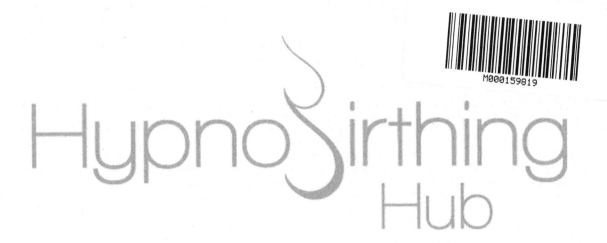

M000159819

Home Study Course Manual

Step by step guide to a natural, easy and pain free birth

Kathryn Clark

DEDICATION

To my beautiful twins, James and Alyssia, who came into the world the most serene way possible. Your birth ignited my passion to share with mothers everywhere the wonder, amazement and magic of an empowering birth.

To my husband John... without your fervent support and your unwavering belief in my ability to make it happen, this program would not have been written. Thank you.

Before you were conceived

I wanted you.

Before you were born

I loved you.

Before you were here an hour

I would give my life for you.

This is the miracle of life.

Maureen Hawkins

CONTENTS

Acknowledgements

There was a time long ago when we women were in tune with our birthing bodies, and we birthed like other mammals. We were calm, relaxed and surrendered willingly to the natural power of our body to give birth to our babies. The instinctive process happened easily, comfortably and quickly. For many women around the world today, this is how they give birth. But for many of today's women, in our 'modernized' culture, birth is mostly akin with pain, fear, medication and disappointment.

There have been many pioneers shouting from the rooftops about better ways of birthing. They blazed the trail, calling that we use our own intuition and innate ability to birth easily. We as a society have only heard faint echoes of whispers of better births and have been deaf to the bellowing shouts.

Thank you, **Dr. Jonathan Dye**, who in the late 1800s wrote the ground breaking book *Easier Childbirth* on natural childbirth 'without pain or peril.' You inspired other pathfinders like **Dr. Grantly Dick-Read** (1890), whose book *Childbirth Without Fear* returned women their rightful gift of a truly natural childbirth.

Franz Anton Mesmer was the first to understand how hypnosis worked. He made special mention of the benefits of hypnosis in childbirth when he stated in 1784 that 'women should not need to suffer pain during childbirth.' His work set the foundation for the hypnosis in Hypnobirthing Hub Home Study Course.

A sincere thank you to those who started teaching hypnosis as a crucial part of childbirth preparation. My gratitude as well to those who coined the phrases 'Hypnosis in Childbirth,' 'Hynobabies,' 'Natal Hypnotherapy,' and most importantly, 'Hypnobirthing.'

I thank **Marie Mongan** for her ground-breaking book written back in1989. Twenty five years ago, she courageously challenged the standard anesthesia and assisted surgical birth.

Thank you to the many hypnobirthing practitioners worldwide who carried the torch in further developing hypnobirthing principles and being passionate about spreading the hypnobirthing word.

A personal thank you to **Hale Dwoskin** *The Sedona Method*, your ideas allowed me find my own emotional freedom. Thank you for the inspiration to develop my own emotional release tools and techniques for pregnancy and birth, found uniquely in the Hypnobirthing Home Study Course.

To the modern day natural birth trail blazers of midwife, **Ina May Gaskin, Dr Michel Odent, Dr Sarah Buckley,** and too many others to list here - you are an inspiration and guide.

To the countless midwives, doctors, obstetricians, and other pregnancy and birth professionals - my deepest thank you for your continued recommendation and support of the Hypnobirthing Hub Home Study Course.

Last, but certainly not least, a heartfelt thank you to the thousands of parents who have entrusted me to shape and guide their most precious birthing day. I am honored and privileged to have shared this transforming experience with you. Thank you.

Preface

So just imagine with me now ...

You are a young woman who has lived her whole life in a small village, in a country only a few hours' flight from your own, and you are pregnant for the first time. For as long as the sun first shone upon your face, pregnancy and birth have been part of your existence. In your village and country, this wonderful stage is a natural expression of love, joy and a connection to life.

As you live closely together, you are comfortable with your body and all its functions. Why shouldn't you be? You have found the freedom to bathe naked in the river while casually chatting to your friends. And have watched and helped as other women have gone into labor and given birth with ease. You have taken part in wonderful rituals of singing and dancing to help the mother achieve a comfortable journey through the giving birth. You have been part of the group that brings special gifts and celebration food after the baby has been born. For centuries, your people have celebrated birth. And now it is your turn.

During your pregnancy, you have been given the best food; you have been massaged and have been the focus of many storytellers. Yet you still work hard, cook food, carry wood, and fetch water. Your body is strong, fit and healthy. And now you are excited and looking forward to a rite of passage, another journey to becoming a mother.

At the same time you know that the birth can take some time. You know that it can be hard work and that your body will release water and blood. You accept that your stomach will go hard and soft, and know that your vagina will open and give way for your baby to be born. Remembering the many other births you have seen, how calm and tranquil the mothers were, even as they knew their bodies were working hard. You look back at the picture of how these mothers about to give birth seemed to be in a different place in their mind. Knowing that you will have the love and support of these women as you embark on the journey they've been through, you can freely surrender to the power and force in your body. You calmly accept that it's your time to bring your baby into the world, and the comfortable process will take place just as you have seen so many times before.

Now take a moment to come back to your reality...

Where are you right now? Is the society or culture the same as the young woman? What do you feel about birth? Is it different from this young woman's feelings? I don't need to tell you that in our present generation and culture, being pregnant and giving birth is far removed from the life and beliefs of this woman. She has many feelings and views of birth, true - But the one emotion which is not present is fear. **She has no need to be frightened**.

Birth is part of life. Everyone eats and everyone goes to the toilet. For the woman, she does marvel at her body. She does not fear it as she does not need to. She has a completely natural and built-in trust and belief that her body will do what it needs to in order to digest food, to breathe air and to give birth.

Yes, she does not understand how her body gives birth, she has not learned about the mechanics of birth, and she has not learned about all the things that can go wrong. Why should she? She has the wisdom and experience of the other women around her to help her if need be. She is, after all, surrounded by women who have seen all kinds of births and who have remedies to help even the hardest birthing situations. She knows that if the baby is long in coming, the women will suggest different ways to stand, different ways to move, and different ways to massage her body. These women around her would readily help the baby into the best position for birth. She has gathered all the learning she needs from being a part of other women's experiences.

In our world, we cannot miraculously recreate the small communal environment where participating in other women's births is acceptable and encouraged. Many of us cannot give birth surrounded by familiar faces in a familiar setting. The 'modernized' world does not see birthing that way.

What you can do.....

But what is in every woman's power is the ability to reconnect with her body's ability to give birth. You can change your beliefs about birth, and you can overcome any fears so that you are more freely able to trust in your body. You can alter the 'modernized' beliefs and methods, and hand over control from your mind to your body's instinctive functions and processes.

More so, you can also share your positive experiences with other women. You can be instrumental in encouraging and teaching them that birth can be a positive and empowering experience. The more that woman share empowered stories about birth, the less other women will see birth as something frightening, painful or hard.

Whatever your experiences are, how your mother gave birth to you, whatever your fears and concerns are about giving life to your baby and where you plan to give birth, there is one lovely truth that will appease your negative thoughts.

This Hypnobirthing course will help you prepare positively for your amazing birth. It will help you embrace and understand the impact that your thoughts and fears can have on your experiences, specifically with your birth experience. This course will help you learn how to clear the path of obstacles and hurdles, and you will free yourself *(predominantly your thoughts)*. Yes, you will achieve such freedom that when the time comes, your mind will no longer interfere with the already setup bodily functions of giving birth.

I challenge you to take this home study course with an open mind, and allow yourself to just entertain the notion that birth is meant to be natural, normal and safe. Most importantly, the most empowering and fulfilling experience in your life will be this birth, and it will stay with you for the rest of your existence.

Let your journey begin...

Introduction

Don't tell my husband, but the best day of my life was not our beautiful wedding day. We were blessed with perfect sunny autumn weather, which formed the ideal backdrop as we said our vows on a white sandy beach in Sydney. Our wedding was lovely, wonderful, in fact. Yet nothing will ever come even close to the day I birthed our twins. This idyllic memory will be etched forever on the landscape of my mind. Even today, some eight years later, the memory still brings tears to my eyes. As I think back and smile, I always relive the joy and excitement of that special day.

Come to think of it, if you ask a 90-year-old woman with Alzheimer's about her births, she will have touching stories to tell about it. With her condition, the near-century-old mother may not remember what she had for breakfast, yet the birth memory is as fresh as if it happened yesterday. Most likely, she will tell of the emotions like sadness, disappointment and regret when she speaks of the birth of her son. Or she would expressively share the emotional high, excitement and love when she fondly re-tells her daughter's birth.

Truth is, we all remember our birthing experiences, and feel the full force of an open floodgate of the emotions that we associate with the experience. We feel these emotions, no matter if that birth experience is a good one or a sad, disappointing one.

Wouldn't it be wonderful if we could ensure that we are more likely to have the emotional highs at birth rather than the lows with our birthing day? Wouldn't it be lovely to remember that such a day is one filled with joy, peace and comfort? With the Hypnobirthing Home Study Course, your birthing dream is not just possible, it is entirely likely!

Over the many years that I have been creating and teaching the Hypnobirthing Hub Home Study Course, we have collected statistics on birthing outcomes. Over 85% of Hypnobirthing Home Study Course mothers birthed naturally and easily, with most saying that they were entirely comfortable throughout the birth and didn't even think of asking for pain medication.

You are reading these words because you have decided to give the best possible birth experience for you and your baby. You are creating a conscious choice to select positive and empowered memories for your birth, and these glorious memories will last a lifetime and become the most treasured of your experiences.

You will come to this hypnobirthing course with doubts, concerns and fears about your ability to birth with ease, naturally and comfortably. Don't worry. It is perfectly normal to feel this way at this time, and it is important to acknowledge how you feel. You may doubt that hypnobirthing actually works at all. Perhaps you're thinking that this method would work for others, but somehow your body or circumstance is different. You may even have gone straight to thinking, *"85% had amazing births, yet I bet I will be in the 15% whose births didn't go as well. I am a magnet for bad luck!"*

It is true that even with the best preparation, some births won't go as planned. In this course, you will learn how to easily focus on the positives, and change your thoughts to believing that you are entitled to have an amazing transforming birth experience. Just like anyone else. Just like any mother-to-be.

By the end of the course, you will look forward to the birthing day or due date with glee and enthusiasm. Your confidence in a successful birthing will be a total transformation from fear to fulfilment. And, of course, that 85% is now securely within your grasp.

Importantly, if your birth happens to fall within the 15%, you now find it easy to be calm and explore your options and make the best possible decision. No matter what happens, you are empowered in your birthing choices. The Hypnobirthing Hub Home Study Course goes to great lengths to clearly explain and provide guidance around which medical choice is best for each birth situation.

All I ask is that you be willing to open your mind and your heart to this transformational birthing method. Allow its intuitive truth to resonate deeply within you.

How to get the most from the course

The Hypnobirthing Home Study Course is made up of this easy-to-follow manual, eight CDs/Mp3 albums and Hypnobirthing video techniques to view. The Hypnobirthing Home Study Course works best with the CD's /Mp3s and the videos, yet this Hypnobirthing manual is fully self-contained.

The Hypnobirthing video techniques: These are free resources and are found on our website: www.hypnobirthinghub.com alternatively, download our free 'Hypnobirthing Video Techniques' App on both iTunes and Android.

Hypnobirthing Hub eight CDs/Mp3 pack: The choice to utilize this pack, is entirely your own. Many women have had amazing Hypnobirths without integrating the CDs/Mp3, yet most have benefited from using all aspects of the Hypnobirthing Course. The Hypnobirthing Hub CDs/Mp3s can be purchased as a pack or each Mp3 is also sold separately on our website www.hypnobirthinghub.com or iTunes or Amazon. Please download a free Hypnobirthing Hub Pregnancy Health and Relaxation Mp3 from **ww.hypnobirthinghub.com/resources**

Unit Integration: At the end of each of the five Hypnobirthing Hub units, there will be:

1.   Unit Summary
2.   Skills builder
3.   How partners can help
4.   Checklist of what you have learnt
5.   Hypnobirthing Mp3s to listen
6.   Hypnobirthing video to watch

Note: **If you are choosing not to listen or view any Hypnobirthing Mp3s or videos, please just ignore these sections in the manual.**

There are 5 units in the manual:

1.   **My body is ready for birth** – An examination of the difference between the natural, calm births of animals compared to the chaotic birthing process women go through. We learn how to prepare our bodies for birth so that it is simpler, calmer and quicker.
2.   **My mind is ready for birth** – Learn how powerful your mind is and how it can be used to create positive or negative results. Discover how to create and sustain positivity in both your visions and your actions. Here we will create the birth picture you most desire, down to the minute details that will make the picture real.
3.   **I have the tools for birth** – A completely relaxed body is the key to a comfortable birth. Discover the deep relaxation triggers, breathing techniques and visualization methods that will enable you to stay in complete control of your comfort levels. This section also gives partners the tools to confidently and calmly support you.
4.   **I have the birth knowledge** – You will find out about the way in which your body was designed to give birth so in most instances there is no need for medical intervention. Should you need to make a decision regarding change in your birthing plan, you will know the very best options for you and your baby.
5.   **I am now completely ready** – A recap and breakdown of the four units and how they are used over the course of your pregnancy. No matter when you start this course, there are practice sections specific for your stage of pregnancy.

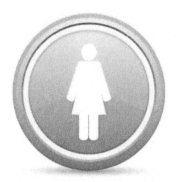

UNIT 1: MY BODY IS READY FOR BIRTH

This unit starts with a snapshot of where you are emotionally with your pregnancy and birth. When you have finished the course, take a look back at this section and see how far you have come. You will be amazed at your transformation!

Later, we explore the easy, calm and instinctive births of animals, and discover the reasons why many women birth so differently. Our modern birthing culture is based on irrational fears and negative beliefs that fundamentally influence our births. We examine how our birthing history shaped the society's thinking.

Next, we move to the important task of preparing our body in pregnancy. With our body ready for birth, the experience becomes easier, quicker and more importantly, we are less likely to need medical intervention.

HOW ARE YOU FEELING ABOUT YOUR BIRTH?

Throughout your pregnancy, the majority of your antenatal care will be focused on the physical well-being of you and your baby. **However, your emotional well-being plays an important part in your approach to pregnancy and birth**. By understanding a bit more about your own feelings, beliefs, hopes and fears, you can begin to separate out those feelings. You can then identify which are useful and beneficial, and know those that are not useful and do not serve a positive purpose.

Before you go on any further, get yourself a pen and spend some time thinking about each of these questions. You can write them here in the book or on a separate piece of paper. However, I would urge you to write them down, as this will encourage you to be focused, specific and conscious about your feelings and thoughts. It will also help you later on if you choose to do the *"Release all Fear of Birth"* exercise and Mp3. Talk to your most quiet, peaceful self... Ask... Then answer by writing it all down. There is no right or wrong answer; only your most honest questions, fears, concerns and issues. Just write it all down.

Remember, this is just a snapshot of where you are right now. Once you have all the tools, resources and understanding that this course provides, you will be amazed at how much more confident, calm and positive you have become about birth. Examining how you feel about pregnancy and birth right now is the first step to accepting - and then letting go of any unnecessary or unhelpful thoughts.

Mother's Thoughts

"After a really terrible experience with my daughter, I was determined to find a different way when I got pregnant this time. My biggest fear came for the old memories which still gave me nightmares at times. I felt sure that the same thing would happen again.

When I did the Hypnobirthing Hub course, there were two things which really stood out for me. First was that I can now see why and when things started to go wrong the last time. If only I had known all of this the first time around. Second, the "Fear Release" exercise made so much difference; they were really powerful. I actually felt the bad memories leave my mind. It did feel a bit surreal. I was able to completely let go of them and they didn't come back, at all. The nightmares also stopped. And with all the other techniques that I had learned, I spent the rest of my pregnancy looking forward to the birth and not dreading it. I think the key thing for me was being completely honest with myself about how I was really feeling about the birth, and not just pushing it all deep down. I know that if I buried it, it would just come back on the day.

I had a wonderful birth. Baby Asha was born peacefully and easily after six hours of labor. None of the old fears came back and I was so pleased how calm, focused, and relaxed I was. I wish every woman around the world had access to these techniques." **Sima Hardy, Suva, Fiji**

YOUR PREGNANCY THOUGHTS

- Was this a planned pregnancy?
- What were your initial thoughts about being pregnant?
- How do you feel now about being pregnant?
- Are you welcoming the changes that are taking place?
- What are three strong emotions that you feel when you think about being pregnant?
- Do you feel you have all the support that you need?
- Other thoughts?

YOUR BIRTH THOUGHTS

- What are your concerns or fears about giving birth?
- Where are you planning to give birth? What are the main reasons for choosing that place?
- Who will be with your during the birth? Why have you chosen them to support you? How well do you think they will support you?
- What was your own birth like? Does your birth affect how you will give birth?
- How have births from friends, family or TV/movies affected your views on birth?
- If you have given birth before, write down any memories, feelings or events that you want to change this time around.
- Have you ever been to a birth? If so, what were your feelings about it?
- In an ideal situation, how would you like the birth of this baby to be?

PARENTHOOD THOUGHTS

- What sort of a parent do you aim you be?
- Could your own childhood affect your ability to be the parent you want to be?
- What sort of parent will your partner be? How do you feel about this?
- What steps will you take to be the best possible parent?

ANIMALS HAVE EASY BIRTHS... SO WHY NOT US?

We have instinctive knowledge to create a child. The DNA within us as women, tells our body how and when to release an egg, how to prepare a safe place for the egg to be fertilized, and the recipe to grow a perfect child. Then the DNA within our growing babies provides all the instructions as to when and how to create brains, lungs, eyelashes, ears and so on. The DNA within us has ensured that the physical structure of our uterus and pelvis is perfectly designed as well. It is structured to change and adapt to accommodate our growing babies. Our female brain and body work in complete harmony, producing all the right hormones throughout our pregnancies and to the birth of our children.

Once our babies are born, our genetic makeup ensures that our breasts can then provide all the nourishment and immunity that our children needs for the first part of their life.

All cells are designed to fulfill a purpose

All the cells in your body have a purpose, and they instinctively know what to do. Look at these processes closely - No one ever taught your body how to digest food or how to fight off a cold. Your heart is continually contracting and releasing twenty-four hours a day. Did you ever have to teach a child how to do a bowel movement?

All of these functions happen painlessly in a healthy body. Yes, if there is damage or a block of energy from things such as stress, fear or bad eating habits, then these functions can become painful or discomforting. In the same way, your body was designed to birth your baby without significant pain. It is only when there is a change from the natural process, such as an induction or an emotional block from things such as fear, tension or anxiety that the birthing process becomes excessively painful.

With such an amazing DNA set-up and such a perfect system, why is it that so many women have lost the belief in their body's ability to give birth?

Essentially, you and I are mammals

We are very sophisticated, clothed and clever, but just mammals nonetheless. Our primal needs and the primal needs of babies are still essentially the same as with other mammals.

Mammals are classified by the fact that a female grows her baby within her body. Like mammals, her brain then secretes a number of hormones that trigger and maintain the muscular movements needed to give birth, and she then provides milk for her offspring once they have been born.

Maybe you have seen wild animals give birth on a nature program, or you have taken a sneak peek at your cat giving birth. Given the right conditions, i.e., an undisturbed natural setting and environment, what are the key characteristics of a mammal's birth experience?

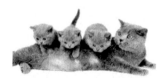

Characteristics of a mammal's birth

- First, they find somewhere safe and quiet, or prepare a relaxed environment for the birthing.
- Mammals usually give birth in the dark.
- As they near birthing, mammals appear very relaxed and calm.
- Mammals appear to be without pain during the process.

Even though we know that animals feel pain in other situations, during the birth they usually remain quiet and calm. As far as we can tell, a mammal does not question what will happen to her during birth. She does not know about the physiological process. She has not watched "Discovery Health" or "One Born Every Minute." She simply accepts what happens to her, does not fight it, and lets her body get on with it. She trusts her body and her instincts.

Mammals influence their own birth

In essence, a mammal will not give birth if she feels that she is in danger, threatened, observed or disturbed. Somehow, a powerful response in her body kicks in to enable her to stop or substantially slow down the labor until she can get somewhere safe and allow the birthing to continue. This is an example of what is known as the "fight or flight" mechanism.

For example, migrating wildebeests will all go into labor and give birth within hours of each other, while the rest of the herd stops and protects the birthing females. In research trials, pregnant chimpanzees that were being observed did not give birth until the researchers gave up waiting and went home.[1]

We can influence our birth as well!

In the same way as other mammals, women also have this instinctual mechanism to shut down or slow down labor if they feel frightened, observed or feel it is not safe to give birth.

Imagine yourself as a woman alone laboring in a jungle. Suppose you saw, or even thought you saw, a fierce animal lurking in the nearby shadows. What do you think would happen? Would you have a conscious choice on what happens next? You may think you could control the situation, but your body would already have made the decision: *your labor would slow down or even stop until you could escape and feel safe again.*

 Mother's Thoughts

"When I read about mammals having great births, I looked at YouTube and typed in "Animal births". I kept clear of the ones that were a bit gory and there was one that was pretty amazing. This elephant in Thailand gave birth and it was wonderful and not a sound! Ever seen an elephant baby? They are pretty big, so I don't think I have anything to complain about. So when the elephant was born, it wasn't breathing and they just let her do what she needed to do and there she was kicking it in the chest to make it breathe, and it did! Wow, it was all ok, and what's more, the vet didn't intervene at all and just let her get on with it.

So every time I have a tiny bit of doubt over my birth, I watch an animal giving birth and feel so much more in touch with nature and my own instincts to birth. I know I can do it! Thanks so much for pointing out such an obvious thing; that animals have easy births without pain, so why shouldn't we? It's starting to make more sense now." **Ava Te Water, Johannesburg, South Africa**

All mammals share the same hormones

The human birth is like that of other mammals, where those animals that suckle their young involve the same hormones: **the body's chemical messengers**. These hormones, which originate in the deepest

---

[1]Newton, N., 1971, Interrelationships Between Various Aspects of the Female Reproductive Role, Psychosomatic Medicine in Obstetrics and Gynaecology, Third Congress.

and oldest parts of our brain (primal brain), cause the physical processes of labor and birth, as well as exert a powerful influence on our emotions and behaviour.

Researchers, such as *French surgeon* and natural birth pioneer *Michel Odent,* believed that if we can be more respectful of our mammalian roots and the hormones that we share, we can have more chance of a straightforward birth ourselves.

Human differences and other mammals

So why is a human mother often perceived to have such excruciating and agonizing pain giving birth when other mammals do not?

One physiological difference is the altered shape of a women's pelvis and birth canal, which over time is caused by our upright stance. Our babies need to twist and turn to navigate these unique bends. Even our nearest cousins, the great apes, have a near-straight birth canal. But even with this difference, a women's body is still able to birth just as easily. The human birthing body just needs a little more time in labor than other mammals.

The main difference between mammals and humans is that we have developed much larger and more **complex brains.** We still have the primal part of the brain, which functions in the same way as those in other mammals, but we have also developed the newer part of the brain called the **Neocortex or "Critical Mind".** It's this part which is responsible for the development of intelligence, analysis, language, inhibitions, and irrational fears and emotions. It is the stimulus to this part of the brain that causes the human mind to "interfere" with the instinctive birthing process, and so lose the ability to completely let go and surrender to the birthing instincts.

At the top of the list of differences between us and mammal are the **emotions of fear and anxiety**. At times, these fears are not truly real, but we feel them as if they are present with us and are part of us. Fear and anxiety can have a real physical impact on the progress and feelings of comfort of all birthing mammals. We will explore how we control and eliminate our fears in detail in Unit 2.

For now, it is important to understand and examine where our fears of childbirth came from and whether these fears are based on fact or folklore.

HISTORY OF FEAR BASED CHILDBIRTH

When a woman gives birth in a supportive environment with the right conditions, birth is an amazing, instinctive and powerful experience. Sadly, this is far removed from the usual media portrayal of women screaming in terror and agony.

Before we go on to look at the impact that these emotions can have on the birthing process, it is useful and interesting to look back in time. It will somehow enable us to understand how women and society have changed from viewing birth as an empowering, enlightening, powerful and natural event to one of which most women are terrified.

How birth was meant to be...

Powerful, strong, healthy & instinctive women

Much of our knowledge about what birth was like in the past comes from traditional birth art, from Stone Age sculptures to statues in ancient Greece, from engravings from Peru to birth art from Native Americans. The majority of art depicts similar scenes, with women in upright positions being supported by other women, and the birthing women are shown as calm, strong and powerful.

Many birth case studies have been documented by early explorers. For example, in 1701, a traveler among the Guiana women in South America noted: *'Women are rarely sick from childbirth, suffer no inconveniences from the same, nor do any die on such occasions'*[2]

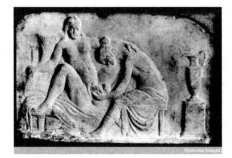

The Ostia Plague Roman Artifact

Women who gave birth using just their instincts and ancient birth knowledge were traditionally **strong, fit and healthy**. They continued to be active throughout pregnancy. By keeping active, strong and fit, the women continually used their bodies and muscles in ways that were helpful later in childbirth. They spent much of their time *squatting* so that their perineal, vaginal and thigh muscles were strong and supple. So then they were able to give birth in positions that were instinctive and supportive to the work of the uterine muscles and birth with gravity.

Birth was in (or near) the home

Birth was often supported by members of a small, close-knit community. During their pregnancy, women were supported by other women they knew and trusted. However, it was always the birthing woman that birthed her baby; she did not have her baby "delivered".

In some cultures, women had special places to give birth, such as the *Baobab tree* for the Hadza tribe in Tanzania, or purpose-built *nesting houses* for the Maori. What is consistent is that women gave birth in a familiar environment and felt supported.

Traditionally, one of the most common positions for women to give birth in is kneeling up and resting their body against a tree or stool. This was referred to in the Bible, by Roman poets, and in birth art from Native Americans.

The wave of change....

As Europe began to develop and move away from the hunter-gatherer lifestyle, communities became larger and ultimately urbanized. This brought with it many changes that contributed to a dramatic shift in the health and well-being of women and the birthing culture.

This urban crowding brought with it a poorer quality of life, increased malnutrition, and spread of disease. Community members experienced drastic changes in their health due to lack of sunlight and exercise, and the unhygienic conditions they live with. In such settings, women were no longer as fit, strong and healthy. And so childbirth brought with it a whole array of complications, which led to a growing fear of the consequences of childbirth. For the first time, it seemed childbirth was something to be feared.

In spite of the industrialization of birth in the modern world, 90% of everyone alive in the world today was born at home.

[2]George J. Englemann, Labor among Primitive Peoples (St Louis MO:JH chambers 1882: reprint New York AMS press).

Advancement of medicine

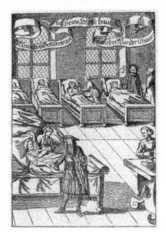

During the Middle Ages and the *Renaissance (the thirteenth to the seventeenth century)*, the early development of medicine had a long-lasting impact on birth culture. **Many countries forbid women from practicing medicine or religion** (often closely linked). During the period, the women who understood how the body worked, used herbs and traditional methods to help women during labor. These who were midwives or healers, were seen as witches and were executed *en masse*. With the execution of these wise women went much of the traditional birth wisdom.

Around that same time, the medical profession was also developing and women were banned from studying or being recognised as professionals in the field in any way. To help with the development of medical learning, hospitals were set up as institutions to give medical students a place to learn and practice their trade.

Hospitals were very different from today

Back then, hospitals were filthy, noisy, crowded places, rife with infection and disease, and there was a serious lack of hygiene. The complications and death rates in hospitals, especially from childbed fever, were extremely high.

It was only in 1847, that a wise man named Dr. Semmelweiss realised that the cause of childbed fever was the lack of hygiene among doctors. It was common for doctors to go straight from dissecting dead bodies to performing internal examinations on birthing women without washing their hands. It was only once it became standard practice in the 1890s for doctors in hospitals to wash their hands between patients that the maternal death rate went down. But by that point, many generations of women had gone into labor feeling petrified of birth, knowing that death was not an unusual outcome for women going into labor.

In addition, during this time, women were no longer encouraged to be upright, but were expected to **lie flat on their back during labor**. It was explained to them as a more convenient position for the doctor to assess how the labor was progressing. As more women gave birth without the traditional love, support and birth knowledge from other women, this added to the increasing numbers of childbirth complications. With all these, it is easy to understand how women became terrified of birth.

Industrialization of birth

By the nineteenth century, most women viewed labor as terrifyingly painful and dangerous. So when the drug *chloroform* was introduced, it was heralded as a major breakthrough in helping women deal with the pain of birth. Queen Victoria was given chloroform in 1853 for the birth of Prince Leopold.

Women who had chloroform were literally knocked out during the birth and would take several days to recover from the effects of the gas. A mother was not conscious to birth her baby and an episiotomy and a forceps delivery was the standard delivery method. As a result, for the first time since human civilization began, babies were routinely taken away from their mothers at a time which is so crucial to the health, well-being and bonding of mother and baby.

From the 1900s onwards, hospitals became cleaner, and giving birth was getting safer. During the process, chloroform took all the pain away. But birth was so far removed from the instinctive natural process. Women at that time did not question any intervention, and they were certainly not in control of their birth experience.

Author's Thoughts

"And while they don't give chloroform today, it was only our mother's and grandmother's generations that had mandatory episiotomies, legs in strips and forceps delivery. I remember my mother telling me of the horror she had when she birthed her first child, my sister. It was 1969 and she was all alone and scared. Husbands weren't allowed in the labor wards at that time. Birthing was 'women's business' and men should be spared the 'trauma of birthing'.

My mother was the first out her friends and sisters to birth and being young without adequate understanding or support at birth, she was rightly terrified. She still remembered: about to deliver her baby, lying flat on her back that suddenly the door swung open and in walked three doctors and twenty trainee midwives. The doctors were giving a detailed lesson in birthing. My mum just lost it and felt so exposed, self-conscious and embarrassed and so her body shut down and refused to birth. Of course the doctors were pleased and this became 'a great opportunity to demonstrate all the tools'.

As you can imagine my mother felt her body taken over and abused. She still says today with strong emotion: 'That doctor was a butcher!' At that time she didn't have the ability to choose her own birth path and destiny. I am so lucky that today, I could birth my twins the way I wish it to be was my birth and I felt truly empowered and fulfilled." **Kathryn Clark**

Quick Exercise: *Think about your mother's birth experiences. How did it shape your thinking about how you would birth? What messages where passed down to you as a young girl?*

Today women are disempowered and don't trust their bodies

Most women today become completely disempowered and no longer trust their natural instincts. Birth has become a medical event which needs to be managed by medical professionals. No wonder that women became so fearful of giving birth!

This is a very depressing and upsetting picture of birth. However, now that you understand where modern birth culture has come from, it will become easier to recognize where many women's fears stem from. The most important thing to remember is that although times have changed and the world around us has moved on, the woman's body and the thousand-years-old built-in process of birthing has not!

As one of the first pioneers to reclaim instinctive birth, **Grantly Dick-Read** wrote in his ground-breaking book Childbirth Without Fear:[3]

'As you understand how deeply and how widely fear has permeated our birth culture and perception of birth; you can still choose to birth fear free, in love and belief that your birth will be a truly empowering and amazing process.'

---

[3]Dick-Read, G.,2003, Childbirth Without Fear, Pinter & Martin.

Wait ... the Bible says birth should be painful?

I wanted to include this account of the history of women and birthing, not to dwell on the negative past, but rather as an explanation of how the social influences of the early centuries caused birthing to go off course. No matter what our religion is (or perhaps isn't), I want women to know how society's evolution left us clinging to a strong belief in the necessity of pain and anguish in childbirth.

My mother still talks about her births. Her words echo through; that births are meant to be painful because the supposed "Curse of Eve." And while she did suffer with each of her four births, on some level she felt she was doing 'God's will' in giving birth in pain.

Even if you have no religious beliefs, just growing up in our society will have ingrained certain thinking on your subconscious mind from such an early age. You may be surprised what you actually believe about pain and birth. Take a moment to fully examine this thinking.

Even though I knew pain and birth did not have to be related, I somehow 'believed' deep down that pain would occur for me because it was 'the natural order of things'. No matter what I learned or did, my births would be painful. I had to work hard on removing that belief and installing a new more empowering, positive belief about birth being comfortable.

For those who can identify with the 'Curse of Eve 'predicament on some level, add it to your 'fears list' (Unit 2) and eliminate it once and for all! I don't think that I would have had the birth of my dreams if I had pushed this hidden belief down and ignored it.

So what does the Bible actually say about birth?

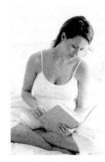

The belief in a curse that made pain part of birthing has more to do with a time in history than biology or observation. However, as we have seen, many people believe that to experience childbirth without pain would be against the word and will of God. According to Helen Wessel, founder of Appletree Ministries and author of *The Joy of Natural Childbirth: Natural Childbirth and the Christian Family,* Hebrew scholars would differ. Wessel states that *"There is no anthropological evidence to support the theological dogma that women of all cultures have universally regarded childbirth as an 'illness' or a 'curse.'"*

We know today, in some of the 'less sophisticated' societies where people haven't been influenced by the views of Western civilization, women give birth with relatively ease and with minimal discomfort. And to think, women's bodies around the world are physiologically the same.

To understand where the 'sorrow' with which women have supposedly been cursed; we need to visit 3000 B.C. It was at this point in history when it was first documented that women had their babies naturally and with a minimum of discomfort, unless there was complication. Wessel cites many references in the Bible which support the blessing of motherhood and the procreation of life. She points to the time of Moses when Jewish women had their babies quite easily and within a relatively short period of time, often without assistance. Historical records of the period just prior to the time of Jesus indicate that births were often accomplished in less than three hours.

Importantly, there were no records of a "curse" having played any part in their beliefs or their birthing. At the end of the second century A.D., however, there arose a widespread wave of contempt against women, and particularly the midwives, healers and wise women who had been so instrumental to birth. Clement of Alexandria wrote: "*Every woman should be filled with shame by the thought that she is a woman."*

The law now demanded that women be segregated during pregnancy and isolated during birthing. As women were labeled seductresses, and all the resulting pregnancies were seen as the product of "carnal sin," a laboring woman was not considered deserving of attention. Even when a birthing process met with a complication, it was against the law to assist a birth. So the birthing mother was isolated, without support or knowledge, and was terrified. Birth then became a feared ordeal.

It was only at this time in history that what is now known as "The Curse of Eve" became embedded into biblical translations. Previously, there was no mention of a curse, except God's curse upon the ground and its implication that humankind would now have to work to survive.

With the new translation, women were to pay the price of original sin, and it was indeed, a high one. Dick-Read learned that the Hebrew word 'etzev,' used sixteen times in the King James I version, is translated to mean "labor, toil and work" So labor is seen to be something more akin to physical effort of farming the land. However, throughout most Bibles, when the same translators referred to childbirth, the word was interpreted to mean "pain, sorrow, anguish or pangs."

Other scholars, too, point out that the prophets made no such reference to pain in their writings on childbirth. Wessel states that there was never an actual curse placed exclusively on Eve. In Genesis, God uses the very same wording in speaking to Adam as to Eve. The translators, though, influenced by the terrible conditions surrounding birth at the time, chose to translate the message delivered to Eve differently.

In the Renaissance and the rebirth of learning, the birthing plight started to improve. Although even with the introduction of chloroform, widely used for all medical procedures, it was denied to birthing women with complications. When it was suggested that pain relief be an option for birthing women, a New England minister responded that to do so *"would rob God of the pleasure of their deep, earnest cries for help."*

 It is really the misguided beliefs of people that are shaping our current belief about birth? So whatever your beliefs may be, take a moment to independently and fully critic those beliefs. Are these views actually are correct? Do you wish to take them into your birthing experience?

Mother's Thoughts

"Re: "curse of eve"- so agree. But you know in the Catholic Church, the actual belief is that Mary, the mother of Jesus, is the "New Eve," which abolished this curse for us. The story continued and we have a choice to trust in what God gives us or to mistrust what God has given us. If we trust in God's true will, we can have comfortable births as he made our body perfectly and loves us and never wants to inflict pain on us. Through our choices, directly or indirectly (individually or through how society functions), we can have the births that God intended for us. All about free will, choice, empowerment through knowledge and trust and support. **Jessica Meksass, Sydney Australia**

THE BIRTH OF NATURAL CHILDBIRTH

If we lived in a village where natural birth was celebrated, embraced and revered, we wouldn't need to do a Hypnobirthing course. Alas, we live in a 'modernized' time which views birth as a fearsome, painful and punishing experience. We have been influenced, or worse, brainwashed, into being terrified of birth and hence we assume the worst. More so, we need to understand and embrace this Hypnobirthing course to alter such negative perceptions about birth.

Hypnobirthing is about learning a new, positive birth experience and 'unlearning' those past experiences. It is also putting ourselves back into the village community by permeating it into our hearts and minds. With that, we can be surrounded by **positive messages of birth** and come to learn that birth is a safe, magical and deeply spiritual experience for us as women.

Hypnobirthing is getting us back to a more fulfilling, empowering time when birth was seen as a true celebration of life. While most of us don't wish to birth in mud huts, or give birth squatting behind a tree on the way to catch a bus, what we can do is take many of the principles of birth from our ancient sisters and apply these to our modern world and lives.

Dr. Grantly Dick-Read was a pioneer of modern natural childbirth in early twentieth century England. At this time, it was standard practice to anesthetize a birthing mother with chloroform and deliver her baby for her. In London 1913, on a windy, rainy night, he changed his views on childbirth forever.

As a young intern in London's White Chapel District, a humble, poverty stricken area in the East End slums, he was called to attend a woman in labor where he discovered his patient in a dim, soaked room from the leaky roof. She was covered only with sacks and an old, dirty skirt. As he began to put the mask over her face and administer chloroform, she refused the drug, which was a first for Dick-Read. So he stood back and watched as she, with little more than gentle breathing, birthed her baby on her own, with no fuss or noise from the mother. When Dick-Read asked why she had refused the relief from pain, she gave him an answer that he never forgot. "*It didn't hurt. It wasn't supposed to, was it, doctor?* "This honest answer, given in a deep East End accent, had a lasting effect on birthing for many decades.

When he next returned to the hospital, Dick-Read was surprised to hear the nurse explain that it was a very boring night, but that things might pick up because the woman in Room 308 might be having some trouble. He had heard those words before, but now it was not something he could easily dismiss. Unless there was a problem, birth was considered boring?

In the coming months, he saw only educated, very affluent women in the London hospital and he watched the agony, pain and terror that they experienced during their birthing time. However, his mind kept drifting back to the poverty stricken East End woman. He mentally compared his present patients with the calm, comfortable woman who birthed with no difficulty and he asked, "Why?" What is it that made all the difference in their birthing experience?

Similar experiences presented themselves to Dick-Read when he was in the service during World War I. On a battlefield in France, a woman nearing the end of her birthing time approached a trench, asking for the field doctor and Grantly Dick-Read, helped her down into the trench. She seemed to ignore Dick-Read and proceeded to give birth, very easily and apparently with no discomfort, just as the woman had on that evening in London. The woman in the trench seemed oblivious to the war that was going on around her. When she had birthed her baby, she simply wrapped it and went on her way once more across the battlefield.

On a different occasion, he encountered a laboring woman, squatting against an embankment and giving birth. Just like the other births, the baby arrived easily. He watched as she waited for some time, holding the baby in her arms and he could see that the umbilical cord still attached to the baby had begun to thin, like a string. Then she started her journey back to her village with her newborn in her arms. Once more, he had witnessed a normal birth and there was nothing wrong with her labor at all.

These births prompted Dick-Read to question his belief about what he had been taught about labor and birthing in general. He was puzzled over what these 'simple women' brought to their birthing that allowed them to birth their babies without the anguish that he was accustomed to seeing from 'more sophisticated' women. In time, he realised the answer lay not in what these 'simple women' brought to their labors, but rather that they didn't bring fear.

From his study came his theory that **when fear is not present, pain is not present**. Fear causes the arteries leading to the uterus to constrict and become tense, creating pain. In the absence of fear, the muscles relax and become pliable, so the cervix is able to naturally thin and open as the body pulsates rhythmically and pushes the baby with ease.

In 1920, Dick-Read wrote a paper spelling out the answer to the question, "What's wrong with labor?" He called his theory the "Fear-Tension-Pain Syndrome." The doctor proposed the cause of tension within the body is primarily fear and in particular in the uterus. This tension stops the natural birthing process, prolonging labor and causing pain. His colleagues thought he was crazy to even entertain the notion that birth can be pain-free. Sadly, his work fell on deaf ears until many decades later.

Endorphins are our body's natural painkillers

Dick-Read was a half century ahead of his time. Although he couldn't put a name to it, he knew from observation that when birthing mothers are relaxed and calm at birth, something wonderful happens which makes for an easier birth.

The body fills with its own natural relaxant. In the mid-seventies it was discovered that this source was a natural analgesic. By studying the way in which opiates work upon the body, researchers discovered that opiate molecules, when locking onto special receptor sites of neurons in the central nervous system, slowed down the firing rate of the neurons. They discovered that if they *decreased* the firing rate of the neurons, it resulted in a *decrease* in the sensation of pain.

A state of calm and relaxation was the missing ingredient that made the *decrease* possible. It was not long before scientists isolated *endorphins* called neuropeptides in the brain and pituitary gland that have an effect 200 times that of morphine. *Endorphins produce a tranquil, amnesiac condition.* The discovery of endorphins validated Dick-Read's suspicions.

This amnesiac state occurs naturally in birth in all mammals as the birthing mother nears the end of her labor. She slips into a tranquil state, goes deeper within and connects to her baby and her birthing body, leaving all the distractions and of the rest of the world behind.

In the fifties, the second printing of Dick-Read's book was published under the title *Childbirth Without Fear*. For the growing number who didn't buy into the generally accepted belief that there is something terribly wrong with labor, he became a hero. Women were starting to be listened to, and many women who gave birth in the '60s experienced absolutely wonderful births.

Dick-Read's teachings became the foundation for two important birthing movements in the twentieth century: the Lamaze Method and the Bradley Method. For over a decade, women were able to birth their babies free of pain with these methods. Unfortunately, the medical establishment decided to host their own versions of the course, and the Lamaze philosophy was undermined. Most hospitals replaced the course name to "Prepared Childbirth" classes, and focused more on medical intervention and pain control.

In 1989, a hypnobirthing movement came onto the birthing scene, bringing with it a return to the belief that every woman has it within her the power to call upon her natural instinct to birth her babies in the peace and comfort that is most similar to other mammals.

My theories are drawn from observation at the bedside of laboring mothers, not in a laboratory. ~ Dr. Grantly Dick Read

Mother's Thoughts

"After a day of mild twinges, I called the hospital to let them know I might be coming later to have my baby. Whilst chatting with the midwife, I had a few more twinges and she said I should come in.

After a phone call to my husband, he made a mad dash home, falling through the front door. He was panicking a bit and I was the calm one. So at the hospital, I was 4 cm, and the 'twinges' were real surges, but they just felt like nothing more than twinges.

However, every time I had a contraction, all I kept thinking about was how I was getting closer and closer to meeting my baby. I kept visualising my older daughter on the shore in my special place, which was a beautiful sandy island holding a baby, and with every surge, I would ride the crest of the wave. It was taking me closer and closer to the two of them.

My husband was amazing with the light touch massage and the prompts; I could actually feel the rush of endorphins through my body. It left me feeling spacey, but so relaxed. The birth was WONDERFUL!! I loved every second of the experience. I made very little noise; I didn't need to, as I wasn't in pain at all.

As soon as she was born, I said 'I want another one'; I didn't want to stop, I was enjoying it all so much!! **Honnie Swithers, Dublin Ireland**

PREPARE YOUR BODY IN PREGNANCY FOR BIRTH

Remember our ancient or village sisters and how they birthed so easily? Well, a large component of an easy birth is making sure your body is ready for birth. These women would walk for long distances to carry water, continue being active with home chores, and tend to the fields. Pregnant women didn't wear a 'warning fragile' sign, but rather, pregnancy was just part of the process of their life. There was not the temptation to sit for long periods of time, slouching on a lounge chair, and using pregnancy as an excuse to avoid exercise.

Quick Exercise: *Take a moment to assess how much exercise you have been doing in your pregnancy? What types of exercise and what do you plan to get your body ready for the birth?*

Regular exercise in pregnancy helps strengthen muscles, promotes energy, improves mood, reduces swelling and bloating, and even aids digestion. Good body mechanics can also improve posture, reduce backaches, and help you sleep better. By exercising in this way, you are preparing your body for an easy birth, and you are encouraging your baby to get into the **optimal position** for birth.

If you are not in the habit of exercising, now is a good time to start – but do so gently. The purpose of exercise during pregnancy is to remain healthy and feel good, not to lose weight. Exercising regularly or participating in some other physical activity throughout pregnancy causes an increased secretion of endorphins, the natural painkillers that are produced by the body. These natural opiates give a feeling of well-being during and after exercise. In addition, they **cross the placenta** and provide pleasant sensations to your baby.

Researchers have found that women who exercise regularly have higher levels of endorphins while exercising than women who exercise only occasionally. In addition, if you are familiar with tapping into these endorphins during pregnancy, it will be much **easier to access them during birth** when they will be needed.

Exercise guidelines and precautions

- Check with your caregiver before participating in any exercise program.
- Never be breathless! If you are out of breath, your baby is likely to be low on oxygen, as well.
- You should always be able to talk as you exercise.
- Pick activities with smooth, continuous movements rather than jerky, bouncy ones.
- Avoid straining and overstretching.
- Stop if you feel pain or experience any other warning signs.
- After twenty weeks of gestation, do not lie on your back when exercising.
- Drink plenty of fluids during exercise sessions or other physical activities.
- Regular thirty minute sessions three times a week is safer than one long weekly session.
- Your pulse should be less than 140 beats per minute.
- Avoid exercising in hot, humid weather.
- Avoid hot tubs, steam rooms or saunas.

After your fourth month of pregnancy, avoid doing exercises on a firm surface while lying on your back. The weight of the uterus can press on your vena cava (the large vein that returns blood to the heart) and reduce your blood pressure. As a result, the amount of oxygen the baby receives is also reduced. This is one of the reasons that birthing on your back isn't advisable.

During pregnancy, the body produces a hormone called **relaxin** which loosens joints and ligaments slightly in preparation for giving birth. This also means it is easier to strain ligaments and muscles during physical activities. So know your limits! However, the benefit of relaxin is that your body will be able to stretch and bend more easily, and you will notice the changes quickly.

Best types of pregnancy exercises

Brisk walking and swimming are the exercises most beneficial to pregnant women. The researchers found that the exercise group in the study experienced less maternal weight gain, but greater infant birth weight and gestational age. They also experienced shorter labors. The women in the sedentary group complained of more discomforts, such as swelling, leg cramps, fatigue, and shortness of breath.

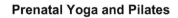

Prenatal Yoga and Pilates

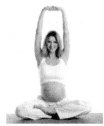

These types of exercises improve muscle flexibility, strength, tone and good posture. And are an excellent way to prepare your body for the work of labor and birth. Women who regularly practice yoga or Pilates reported less back pain, other common discomforts of pregnancy, and, importantly, more babies in the best position for birth. Join a class or check out the many pregnancy Pilates and yoga DVDs, or many YouTube videos are readily available.

Birth ball benefits

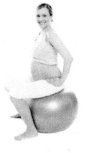

Simply by sitting and rolling with the ball encourages rhythmic movement and pelvic mobility. The softness and shape of the ball absorbs your weight and helps to prevent and relieve back strain. Also kneeling forwards over the ball takes the weight off your back and is great practice for labor. As the ball is not flat, it is always moving slightly as so by sitting on the ball, you will be using your inner thighs and pelvic floor muscles without even noticing. Natural movements with the ball help to gently tone your internal and external pelvic muscles. Many other standard exercises can be done with your birth ball, however ensure you are well balanced. Also sitting on the ball at your desk raises your hips higher than your knees. This encourages your baby to settle into an optimal position for birth.

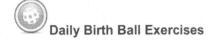

Daily Birth Ball Exercises

- *Sit for at least fifteen minutes per day (great for watching TV or on the PC).*
- Sit with your legs wide apart as you can, you are then easily stretching your inner and outer thighs and opening your pelvis.
- Roll your hips around in a circle, like doing the hula hoop. Move your hips side to side. This exercise is amazing at strengthening most your body in a simple movement.

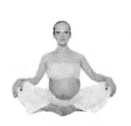

Wall Squat Benefits: Strengthens muscles of the abdomen and thighs, helps to widen pelvis for birth.

Directions: With your back to the wall, with your feet hip width apart. Place your hands on your thighs and press your back and hips against the wall. Slide your torso down the wall until your thighs are almost parallel to the floor (sitting position). Hold for as long as comfortable. Slide back to a standing position.

Frequency: Five repetitions (three minutes)

Caution: To prevent strain on your knees, do not bend past the sitting position. They should not extend over your toes.

Tip: Do this with a birth ball behind you for support and ease.

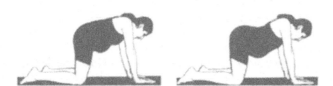

Pelvic Tilt Benefits: Improves postures, relieves back discomfort and pelvic congestion, and increases abdominal muscle tone.

Directions: Kneel on the floor on your hands and knees. Align your head with your spine. Tuck in your buttocks, pull up your abdominal muscles, and press your spine up towards the lower back just enough to erase the spinal curve. Hold as long as comfortable, then return to the starting position. Repeat this exercise using a constant rhythm and rocking motion.

Frequency: Five repetitions (three minutes)

Labor: Helpful to perform in labor as it helps reduce back discomfort in labor.

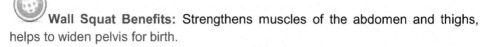

Leg Press Benefits: Stretches the ligaments and muscles of the inner thighs and increases their elasticity for birthing.

Directions: Sit on the floor with the soles of your feet pressed together and pulled toward your body. Using only the muscles of your legs, press your knees downward and hold

Frequency: Five repetitions (three minutes)

Caution: Discontinue the exercise if you feel pain around your pubic bone, which may indicate some separation at the joints. See a pregnancy chiropractor or pregnancy physiotherapist.

 Leg Stretch Benefits: Stretches the ligaments and muscles of the inner thighs and increases their elasticity for birthing. Also stretches the muscles of the lower back and calves.

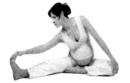

Directions: Sit on the floor with one leg stretched out in front of you as wide as comfortably possible. With the other leg tucked in, lean forward over the straight leg and reach each hand to its corresponding ankle. Repeat with both legs.

Frequency: Five repetitions (three minutes)

Caution: Discontinue the exercise if you feel pain around your pubic bone, which may indicate some separation at the joints. See a pregnancy chiropractor or pregnancy physiotherapist.

Mother's Thoughts

"I had a horror of a first birth. I can't tell you just how much pain I was in and how I just felt traumatised by the whole experience. I still have flash backs where I see the birth all over again. They say you always remember your birth, no matter what it was like, and I do! I hadn't done a hypnobirthing course or anything, but I firmly believed in the body being able to birth on its own. So, I felt I was prepared for natural birthing.

Yet, now as I am about to have my second child and just finished the Hypnobirthing Home Study Course, I can see that I forgot about one absolutely vital thing - and that is making sure my body is up for birth. I know my mind was there, but the body just wasn't following!

My first was in a posterior position and it hurt like hell! With the baby's head turned the wrong way, my body was going in overdrive with contractions for two weeks. And that was even before I started the real labor. My midwife said if a baby settles in a posterior position, it means my body is just doing all it can to stretch my ligaments and pelvis to make sure I can birth. It is just my body doing its job. So two weeks of painful pre-labor, I was so over this and opted for epidural when the real thing came and of cause that meant it all spiraled downhill from there.

Anyway, the killer thing is that I now know that posterior births are mostly in our Western world and all I went through may have been avoided. It does bring a tear to my eye as thinking about how it could have been. Anyway, positive thinking and all that, and I'm now looking forward to my daughter's birth. She is in a perfect, yes, perfect (I scream and tell everyone!) position for birth. All my body preparation is working.

I used to be a bit of a slob, using pregnancy as an excuse for not getting up of the couch. Now, I've just come back from an hour fast walk and finished off with sitting on my exercise ball. I know this birth is going to be wonderful, I feel I am fully prepared now, mind, and body. Thanks so much for showing me a different way of birthing and knowing that this birth will be a transforming and wonderful experience for me. Thanks" **Julie McIntyre, Amsterdam, Netherlands**

YOUR PROPER BODY MECHANICS

The term "body mechanics" refers to the way you use the different parts of your body to move. During pregnancy, moving your body properly is especially important as it helps minimize discomfort as your body gets larger and changes shape.

Standing tall

Good posture is essential throughout pregnancy because your center of gravity changes. As your abdomen grows, you will be tempted to compensate for this change by slumping when you stand. Consciously maintain the same good posture you had before becoming pregnant.

Standing erect helps **prevent or alleviate back discomfort**, improves digestion, and also helps the baby settle into the **optimal birth position**. Women who have good posture during pregnancy are much less likely to have a baby settle into a breech or posterior position. If you are having trouble with your posture, see a pregnancy chiropractor or physiotherapist as soon as possible, and they may need to make a few adjustments get everything aligned.

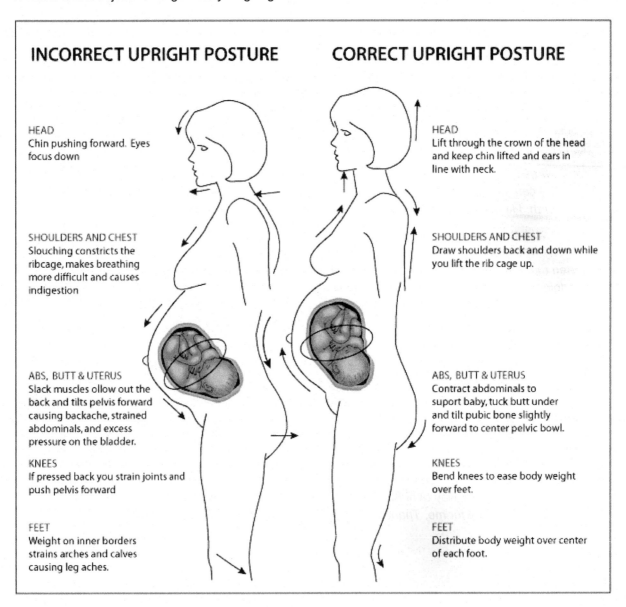

INCORRECT UPRIGHT POSTURE   CORRECT UPRIGHT POSTURE

HEAD
Chin pushing forward. Eyes
focus down

SHOULDERS AND CHEST
Slouching constricts the
ribcage, makes breathing
more difficult and causes
indigestion

ABS, BUTT & UTERUS
Slack muscles ollow out the
back and tilts pelvis forward
causing backache, strained
abdominals, and excess
pressure on the bladder.

KNEES
If pressed back you strain joints and
push pelvis forward

FEET
Weight on inner borders
strains arches and calves
causing leg aches.

HEAD
Lift through the crown of the head
and keep chin lifted and ears in
line with neck.

SHOULDERS AND CHEST
Draw shoulders back and down while
you lift the rib cage up.

ABS, BUTT & UTERUS
Contract abdominals to
suport baby, tuck butt under
and tilt pubic bone slightly
forward to center pelvic bowl.

KNEES
Bend knees to ease body weight
over feet.

FEET
Distribute body weight over center
of each foot.

Courtesy of completeworxmassage.com

Standing technique

- Think tall! While standing, the way you hold your head influences the position of the rest of your body. If you let your head hang forward, your body will droop like a wilted flower.
- Hold your head up with your chin tucked in and your neck straight.
- Imagine there is a piece of string pulling the top of head up and everything is in a straight line.
- Lift your shoulders up and pull them back. This position will keep you from cramping your rib cage, which can make breathing difficult and possibly cause indigestion.
- Pay special attention to your pelvic area which contains the weight of the growing baby. Think of your pelvis as a bowl filled with liquid.
- To prevent the liquid from spilling out, tilt the "bowl" back by tightening your abdominal muscles and tucking your buttocks under. This position prevents excess tension in the lower back muscles.
- To help maintain proper pelvic alignment, bend your knees slightly and keep your body weight over your feet. Balance yourself on the center of each foot, never on the inside.
- When standing for long periods, place one foot on a small stool to flex the hip. This reduces strain on the ligaments in the groin.
- When walking, maintain all of the aspects of good posture. When taking steps, bring your legs straight forward from the hip. Do not swing them sideways in a "waddle."

Sitting straight

While sitting in a chair, sit up straight! Use the back of the chair as a guide to sit up straight. For this reason, straight-back chairs are preferred over cushioned ones during pregnancy. Place a pillow behind your neck and/or the small of your back for increased comfort. The full length of your thighs should rest on the seat, which should be high enough to keep your knees even with your hips.

Sitting in a cross-legged position on the floor, called tailor sitting, is excellent during pregnancy. In addition to being comfortable, it improves the circulation in the legs, while stretching and increasing the flexibility of the inner thigh muscles. Sit this way whenever possible when watching television, reading the newspaper, or folding the laundry. If your legs become tired, stretch them out in front of you.

It has been found that during pregnancy, those women who spent long time in unsupported positions, such as lying or sitting on a sofa, or sitting in a car were much more likely to have their babies in the challenging 'posterior' position for birth. Posterior births are not common in developing countries where daily exercise and correct sitting is usual.

Lying down

Lying flat on your back, the supine position, for extended periods of time is not recommended after the fourth month of pregnancy. This is because the increasing weight of the baby and the uterus will compress your vena cava, the major blood vessel that returns blood to the heart. This can lower your blood pressure, which in turn, will reduce the amount of blood travelling to the placenta and the baby. Refrain from doing any exercises that require you to lie on your back. So at four months, switch to pregnancy specific exercise classes which encourage the correct laying and sitting positions.

Chiropractor Thoughts

During pregnancy your body undergoes great change, especially your spine. As your baby and belly grow your spine adapts its shape by arching the low back, your hips tilt forward and your head and neck move forward also to help establish your balance. These along with your hormonal changes causing ligament laxity, mean that there is a lot more pressure and instability of your low back, pelvis, upper back and neck. The goals of chiropractic care throughout pregnancy are to safely ease your discomfort and help promote a more stable pelvis. As a result chiropractic care has been shown as a way to significantly reduce labor time for women who have care throughout their pregnancy.

In one study, Dr. Joan Fallon found that first-time moms averaged a 24% shorter labor, while experienced mothers (those who had given birth before) had a 39% reduction in the average labor time in a substantial percentage of births. Also by using a specific chiropractic analysis and adjustment known as the 'Webster Technique' enables chiropractors to establish balance and reduce uterine and ligament stress in a pregnant woman's pelvis which makes it easier for a breech baby to turn naturally.

Dr. Wendy Froyland, Chiropractor and Acupuncturist

PELVIC FLOOR EXERCISES

Pelvic floor exercises are designed to strengthen the pelvic floor muscles, which support the bladder, as well as the uterus, urethra, and rectum. By performing pelvic floor exercises regularly during pregnancy, you can achieve voluntary control of the pelvic floor. This will enable you to relax the area consciously during birth. Relaxed pelvic floor muscles will allow your baby an easier passage and perhaps eliminate the need for an episiotomy.

Well-toned pelvic floor

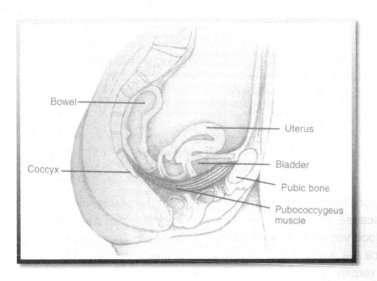

Poorly toned pelvic floor

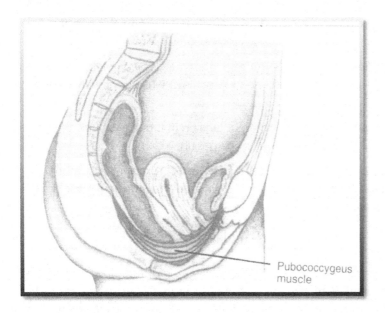

Pubococcygeus
muscle

Birth can affect your pelvic floor

During birth, these muscles are stretched, which can result in a prolapsed (sagging) uterus, a prolapsed bladder, and/or urinary stress incontinence (uncontrolled urine leakage caused by coughing, sneezing, and running, laughing, or jumping). Performing pelvic floor exercises during and after pregnancy can help prevent such problems. When done shortly after birth, pelvic floor exercises help restore the muscle fibers that were stretched during birth.

The benefits of pelvic floor exercises are not limited to the period of giving birth. They extend into the immediate postpartum period and can continue throughout life. Performing pelvic floor exercises helps improve the muscle tone of the vagina, causing it to become tighter, snugger. (Your partner will also appreciate this extra snugness.) It also enhances nerve ending response, resulting in heightened vaginal sensitivity during intercourse.

Locating your pelvic floor

Before performing pelvic floor exercises, you must first locate the pelvic floor muscles. Do this by contracting the muscles around the urethra, as if you were trying to hold back urine.

Next, at a time when your bladder is full, start to urinate and then stop the flow. Do this a few times. Stopping the flow tightens the pelvic floor as releasing the flow relaxes it. Only do this to locate your pelvic floor, not to practice the exercises. Instead, practice them when your bladder is empty.

 Super pelvic floor exercises

While standing, contract the pelvic floor by lifting and tightening the muscles and holding for a **count of twenty seconds**. (Make sure you are doing this without tightening your buttocks or squeezing your legs together, use only your pelvic floor muscles.) Maintain the tension. If you feel the muscles relaxing, tighten them again. **Perform one repetition of this exercise ten times twice a day.**

Lift pelvic floor exercises

This is another variation of this exercise will help you achieve deeper muscle control in preparation for the actual birth of your baby.

To perform this exercise, envisage your pelvic floor as a Lift. Contract the muscles upward from the first floor to the fifth floor, stopping at each floor and increasingly tightening the muscles as you go higher. Then gradually relax the muscles as you move downward from the fifth floor to the first, releasing a little tension at each floor.

Continue moving downward to the basement level where you relax the muscles completely by giving them a slight push. This is the degree of relaxation you will need to achieve while gently assisting the baby down the birth canal.

Always return to the second level to maintain a constant degree of tension in the pelvic floor, the same way that a hammock returns to its normal, higher position when you get up.

With continued practice, you should develop **enough control to go to ten floors**. Make sure that you breathe normally. As your pelvic elevator moves upward and downward, do not hold your breath. **Practice this exercise at least twice a day**.

Practicing tips

Since it is best to perform pelvic floor exercises on an empty bladder, get into the habit of doing just one while washing your hands after urinating. After the baby comes, doing a super pelvic with every nappy change will ensure plenty of practice. Keep in mind that you should practice pelvic floor exercises for the rest of your life, not just while you are pregnant.

 Make pelvic floor exercises apart of your daily routine, by linking this exercise to cleaning your teeth morning and night. It is a time when you are standing and can concentrate.

Mother's Thoughts

'My pelvic floor was tight! It ought to be, I practiced constantly! I was determined to have an easy birth and just do the 'Birth Breathing'. It worked! I relaxed my 'pelvics' during birth and it only took a few minutes for my boy to be born. No suction cup head or salad tongs for him!' **S. Dossetor, Windsor,UK Australia**

PERINEAL MASSAGE

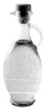 Just as you prepare your muscles for birthing by toning them through exercise, you also need to prepare your perineum. The perineum is the area between the vaginal opening and the anus. It must be readied for the stretching required to accommodate the baby's head. Perineal preparation is especially important if you want to avoid an episiotomy, as preparing the perineum increases the chance of keeping it intact during delivery.

Prenatal preparation of the perineal area begins with good nutrition. Eating properly will contribute to healthy tissues that stretch and heal rapidly. Practicing pelvic floor exercises, waiting for 'your urge' to birth your baby, and do birth breathing. These will help you gain additional control over the perineal area which is very important during your birthing time. Perineal massage will prepare you for the stretching sensations that you will feel during your baby's birth. It also increases the elasticity of the perineal tissues.

Begin perineal massage around thirty-five weeks

You can either do this yourself or have your partner do it for you. It's important that whoever performs the massage has clean hands and short fingernails. For lubrication, you can use a little K-Y jelly, some vitamin E, or olive oil. Some women find that taking a warm bath prior to the massage is helpful. You may want to use a mirror when massaging the area, especially the first few times, for optimum vision.

Practice Perineal Massage three times per week from thirty-five weeks until birth. This will ensure your perineum is stretched prior to birth. It is not necessary to stretch your perineum now to accommodate a baby's head (about ten centimetres in circumference). At the time of birth, the hormone relaxin will help the perineum to stretch as much as needed without tearing. You are just giving your body a helping hand to make it easier for birthing to occur. Also, it will go back to normal once more after the birth!

     The skin of our perineum is able to stretch more than any other part of our body. We are not designed to tear in birth, but rather nature enables our perineum to stretch during birth. So performing perineal massage gives nature an extra helping hand.

Perineal massage technique

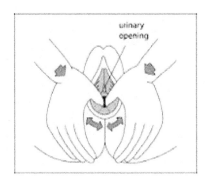

1. To perform the massage yourself, insert your thumbs about three centimetres into your vagina

2. Press your thumbs toward your anus.

3. With your thumbs, slowly stretch your perineal tissues outward toward your thighs. (To begin with, keep the knuckles of your thumbs together to prevent overstretching).

4. You should feel a slight stinging or burning sensation.

5. Continue to maintain this pressure for two minutes, until the perineum becomes somewhat numb and the tingling is less distinct.

6. Then gently slide the tips of the thumbs back and forth as you continue to stretch the tissues outward. Continue this action for another couple minutes.

If you have a scar from a previous episiotomy, spend additional time massaging vitamin E oil into the scar tissue.

Tip: For those want an alternative to Perineal Massage, products such as 'Epi-no' http://www.epi-no.com.au/ have an easy to use pelvic floor trainer and a balloon devise that is inserted into your vagina to stretch the perineal tissues for you. (Epi-no is not sold in the United States).

 Midwife's Thoughts

'There really is such a difference in tearing between those who do perineal massage techniques and those who don't. I wish all women did their homework! Also, it's a mind game situation. Mums, who have this technique down pat, are much more confident in their body and ability to birth easily.' **Belinda Cameron, Midwife US**

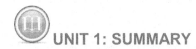

UNIT 1: SUMMARY

- Be totally honest with yourself about how you feel about your birth, pregnancy, and parenthood. 'You can't heal what you can't reveal.'
- Animals have amazing births - you can have one as well! Just trust your instincts like animals do and keep at bay your Neocortex or the 'thinking part' of your brain.
- Our history gave us a flawed view of birth. Look further back into history and discover your own inner ancient birthing women, and bring your empowered birthing into reality.
- Confident, relaxed and centred women around the globe today and in our past have birth easily because fear was absent at their birth. Fear causes pain and intervention. Set yourself free of fear and embrace your innate birthing ability.
- Preparation of your body is vital to your success in birthing. So, become strong, healthy and flexible, just like our tribal birthing sisters. Embrace the new energy and power knowing your body is ready for an easy and safe birth.

Partners can help

- Address your pregnancy, birth and parenting concerns. You are in this together and your thoughts and feelings will affect your partner's confidence.
- Exercise with her. Walking is great, even greater when you hold her hands.
- Buy two exercise balls and both sit while watching TV.
- Do the heavy lifting and other taxing home chores.
- Discourage her from exercise on hot, humid days or find a cool place to exercise.
- Compliment her on her good posture.
- Remind her to do her Pelvic Floor exercises.
- Discourage her from using hot tubs, saunas or steam rooms.
- Offer to give her massages (including perineal massage).
- Treat her to a professional pregnancy massage.

My body's prepared for birth: checklist

- ☐ Regular thirty minute exercise sessions three times a week.
- ☐ Pregnancy Yoga or Pilates at least once a week.
- ☐ Sit and exercise on birth ball for at least fifteen minutes per day.
- ☐ Wall squats three minutes three times a week.
- ☐ Pelvic rock three minutes three times a week.
- ☐ Leg stretch three minutes three times a week.
- ☐ Leg press three minutes three times a week.
- ☐ Sitting correctly with a supported chair or cross legged.
- ☐ Consciously correcting your posture when standing and walking.
- ☐ Pelvic Floor Exercises: twice per day.
- ☐ Practice Perineal Massage 3 x week from 34 weeks until birth
- ☐ I am eating well, giving good nutrition to my baby

Unit 1: Hypnobirthing Home Study Course Recordings

Pregnancy Relaxation and Health

T1 Introduction
T2 Pregnancy Relaxation and Health

T3 Quick Relaxation and Baby Bonding
T4 Pregnancy Affirmations

Listen at least once a week from now until the birth of your baby. By listening to this recording regularly, it will provide the best possible pregnancy experience for you and be a simple reminder for continued health and relaxation during your pregnancy. *To get this free download, please go to www.hypnobirthinghub.com/resources*

Audio Guide – Unit 1 (Track 1)

This guide comprises of additional material to support Unit 1 of Hypnobirthing Home Study Course. You can listen once, or as many times as you need. The audio guide is the only recording that you can listen to while you are driving in the car. **Podcast:** *For this free audio track on this unit, go to http://hypnobirthinghub.podbean.com/ (Episode 1).*

Kathryn Clark's Twin Birth Story

Watch this short video on my own Hypnobirthing experience of bringing my twins into the world and find out why I am so passionate about Hypnobirthing. *www.hypnobirthinghub.com/about*

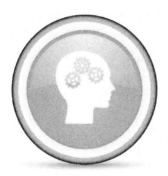

UNIT 2: MY MIND IS READY FOR BIRTH

This part of the Hypnobirthing Hub Home Study Course is about your mind and how it can help or hinder you at your birth. The thoughts you think, the emotions you feel, and the daydreams you visualize all fit together like an intricate puzzle to form your birth picture. So decide now what your birth picture will look like, as every thought, feeling and belief is making a piece of your puzzle. You have the power to create the birth of your dreams by choosing each and every intricate piece of your birth picture.

THE HYPNOSIS IN HYPNOBIRTHING

Now let's look at why we use hypnosis in our Hypnobirthing course.

Simply put, hypnosis enables us to think new, more positive thoughts and expectations about birth. It can also replace more negative thoughts and fears about birth, so we start to automatically think about birth in a positive way. The thoughts that used to get us down and worried just won't be there anymore. It is like a large weight has been lifted off of our shoulders and with this weight removed, we will start to feel confident that the birth of our dreams is in our reach.

I can say one hundred times; *'You are going to have an amazing birth'*. And every time I say this, you process the information and make a critical judgment about it. You can either accept what I said or you can reject it. This **critical reasoning** helps us think independently, build intelligence, and reduce our gullibility. So our critical thought is a good thing and sets us apart from other animals who respond more to instinct rather than critical thought.

However, in birthing we know that humans perform best when we respond more like our mammal cousins. We do so by using our instincts and avoiding too much analysis of the birthing situation. **In hypnosis we easily tap into the more primal and instinctive parts of ourselves.** By being in a deeply relaxed state, hypnosis enables us to temporarily bypass our critical thinking and go straight to **our inner mind**. This access to the deepest part of our mind enables us to more easily accept and welcome new, more positive suggestions and beliefs about birthing.

Again, if I say *'You are going to have an amazing birth'* until I am blue in the face, you may not ever believe me, and so it would be a very short course. Yet with hypnosis, if you are even just hoping to have a great birth experience, your inner mind will be open and willing to accept the hypnotic suggestions.

These suggestions in the entire Hypnobirthing Home Study Course recordings are carefully created to **install more positive beliefs and expectations about birth**. Therefore in time if you are choosing to listen to any of these recordings, you will find that your beliefs and thoughts about birth have changed for the better.

You are now not just '*hoping to have a great birth experience*'. The **'hoping'** has changed to a **'*knowing*'** that you will have a great birth. That is the power of hypnosis, to positively change our thoughts and beliefs at a deep level. Therefore we can become whole, feel free, empowered, and confident with our life.

There are over 1,000 research studies on hypnosis and hypnotherapy cited on PubMed, the world's largest database on scientific research.

Will I remember my birth if I'm hypnotized?

When you are in hypnosis during your birthing time, you'll be able to hear conversations and may or may not wish to join in. Though you will be totally relaxed, you will also be fully in control. For a person who is not familiar with **self-hypnosis**, you may even appear as though you've taken some kind of medication to put you into this profoundly relaxed state. During your birthing, you will be aware of your surges (contractions), but you will experience them comfortably, with the knowledge that you are very much in charge. You'll be able to interrupt your relaxation whenever you wish and resume it whenever you choose.

As you progress closer to birthing, you most likely choose to go to a **deeper level of hypnosis**, to work with your birthing body and your baby, so that together you can work in harmony through birth. Although you can't see your baby at this time, you will be able to physically know that your baby is very much a birth partner in this adventure.

When you are tuned into your body through hypnosis, you will sense and know exactly what you and your baby are doing. You'll become skilled in using your own natural abilities to bring your mind and body into perfect harmony. In addition, the deep **relaxation triggers and techniques** will enable you to connect and work with your body and your baby during your birthing time. The repetitive practice of these techniques will make it possible for you to instantly achieve this relaxation and maintain it for as long as you choose through your birth.

The value of self-hypnosis comes from learning to reach that level of mind where the suggestions effectively influence your physiological birth experience. The daily practice of Hypnosis are vital in conditioning you to a deeper level of relaxation and calm that is needed for your birth. Simply put, **hypnosis is obtaining a deep level of relaxation**.

If you are **willing to apply the practice e** that is required to reach these levels of relaxation, then your birth will be one of ease, comfort and joy. These skills will be applicable to many areas of your life, as well as for the birthing of your child. Parents to be find that the months of preparation in relaxation benefit everyday situations.

Dad's Thoughts

'I came to hypnobirthing to learn the best way to have a baby; instead, I came away with the best way to lead my entire life. I am so grateful for the skills I learned. I even used the relaxation triggers and visualizations to ace an interview and get the job I wanted. I was cool as a cucumber during the interview...I didn't even recognise myself." **Julian Trust, Newcastle, Australia**

HYPNOSIS THROUGH THE AGES

Hypnosis has been used in almost all cultures over time. Over 4,000 years ago, the founder of Chinese medicine, Wang Tai, used words as healing tools, while Druids used 'magic sleep'. Hieroglyphics on Egyptian tombs show sleep chambers as healing centres. Suggestions of the use of hypnosis appear many times in the Bible. It has been argued by biblical scholars that many miracles which happened "within" people can be attributed to the use of hypnotic language to install new beliefs and expectations.

> *During labor, many women instinctively use their imagination to "go to" a safe place in their mind. The place may stay the same or it may change throughout the birthing. Your mind becomes very creative and you may be surprised at the images that your mind creates.*

Hypnosis in our culture

It was the work of Scotsman James Esdaile which is most impressive as the origin of modern hypnosis. Esdaile recorded using **hypnosis as a form of anesthesia** in over 2,000 minor and 300 major operations, including nineteen amputations by 1909.[4] By as early as 1892, the British Medical Association first recognised the use of hypnosis as a therapeutic agent. However, with the introduction of chloroform at a similar time, the popularity of hypnosis as an anaesthetic began to decline. Also around this time, the use of hypnosis took a different turn when it was used to help deal with **emotional and psychological issues** by leading figures such as Sigmund Freud, the founder of psychoanalysis.

THE HISTORY OF HYPNOSIS IN BIRTH AS A PAIN RELIEF

Interestingly, hypnosis for childbirth has been used more formally for over 100 years, with many examples of its use across the world. In the 1920s in the former USSR, the hypnosis pioneer Platonov became well known for his hypno-obstetric successes.[5] These methods using relaxation and hypnosis were later developed by Fernand Lamaze, who created the Lamaze birthing technique. Obstetrician Dr. Joseph B. Delee said in the 1930s that hypnosis was the ***"only anesthetic without danger"*** and told his profession:

"I am irked when I see my colleagues neglect to avail themselves of this harmless and potent remedy. Hypnosis is an effective method of relieving pain in birth without altering the normal course of labor."

Since the 1960s, in the US, UK and Australia, there has been an increase in the use of hypnosis in obstetrics, with many doctors and hypnotherapists supporting, endorsing and practicing the techniques. For example, Dr Werner delivered over 6,000 babies using chemical anesthesia. But when he discovered hypnosis, he went on to support over 3,000 women to give birth using the method.

It was predominantly the work of Dr. Milton Erickson in the USA in the 1950s which changed the medical opinion of hypnotherapy and so helped to legitimize its wide applications in 1955. The use of hypnosis as a form of pain relief was once again recognised and approved by the British Medical Association, which stated that:

---

[4]Milne Bramwell, J., 1909, 'Hypnotism and Treatment by Suggestion', London, Cassell

[5]Gerard V. Sunnen, M.D., 1999, 'Miscellaneous Medical Applications of Hypnosis' Bellevue Hospital and New York University.

"Currently, hypnosis is used and applied in a wide variety of areas, from dealing with post-traumatic stress to overcoming phobias and curing obsessive-compulsive disorders."

This support of hypnosis was closely followed by the approval of the American Medical Association in 1958, the Australian Medical Association, and other medical associations around the globe.

Franz Anton Mesmer was the first to understand how modern hypnosis worked. He made special mention to the benefits of hypnosis in childbirth, when he stated in 1784 'women should not need to suffer pain during childbirth.'

So what exactly is hypnosis?

Despite of the long and credible history of hypnosis, many people today have unpleasant perceptions about it. For them, the term "hypnosis" brings to mind all kinds of images, from swinging pendulums to people acting like chickens on stage. There are many misperceptions of what hypnosis is and what it is not about. However, as more research is done into the benefits of hypnosis there is growing acceptance and awareness of the **connection with our thoughts and the way our bodies function.** As a result, hypnosis is being recognised and is gaining credibility.

Firstly, **hypnosis is a completely natural state of being**. In fact, you have already experienced it thousands of times. It's simply a pleasant state of mental relaxation, during which you are still aware of what is going on around you, but have mentally "gone somewhere else" or "are away with the fairies". The phrase "the lights are on but no one's home" comes to mind.

In these examples, you were not asleep or under the control of someone else, but in your own hypnotic state. You were still conscious and able to function, but your mind had drifted off to thoughts unconnected to the activity you were doing. That is to say that there was a degree of communication between the two different parts of your mind, which we will call the **conscious and the subconscious (or inner mind).**We naturally dip in and out of these two parts hundreds of times a day, so there is always communication between them.

You are hypnotized every day

Being in a hypnotic state is simply a time when you have some or all of the following:

1. You are deeply relaxed

2. You are very focused on one thing

3. Your mind "wanders"

4. You feel a bit distanced from your actual surroundings

5. Time passes in an illogical way

6. You become open to positive suggestions

As you can now see, everyone enters into the state of hypnosis many times a day. You may find you are in a hypnotic state when you have a shower and just alone with your thoughts.

Have you ever seen the faces of the people waiting for an elevator? They seem to be devoid of any signs of life, yet they are simply in a hypnotic state. Have you ever driven your car to work or a familiar place day after day? Then when you have arrived at your destination, it seems your body overtook the journey while your mind was elsewhere? Or perhaps you remember your teacher at school calling your name several times before you 'came back to the room'? These are all normal, natural and every day examples of hypnosis that we all experience regularly.

The **benefits of being in a hypnotic state** are immeasurable and include lower blood pressure, increased energy and a better-functioning body. The state also provides calmer thoughts, better sleep and the ability to deal with situations more effectively.

In our modern society, we hardly ever allow ourselves the time out to get into a hypnotic, relaxed state, and so often our bodies begin to suffer, which leads to a drastically rising rate of stress-related illnesses.

Hypnosis allows access to our subconscious mind

Hypnosis allows us to actively communicate between the conscious and subconscious with a particular purpose in mind, such as preparing our mind to believe that we will have an amazing birth.

A definition by Alman and Lambrou states that: *"While in hypnosis, one suppresses the power of the conscious criticism. During this heightened focus and awareness, suggestions appear to go directly into the subconscious... You can control areas yourself that are normally out of reach of your conscious mind."[6]*

Why do we need two types of minds?

It can be confusing thinking that we have different types of minds in our head, and at times it does seem as if there is a battle going on within us. We have our **'self-talk'** that just seems to pop up in our head and give unwarranted appraisal of our actions. Then we have the quiet inner voice or **conscious** that tells us what is right or wrong.

Ever had an argument, and during the argument you could hear your 'self-talk' telling you, 'to let loose because you are right'? Then later on, in the quiet stillness, you hear a different voice that whispers you were wrong to argue that way? No, you are not suffering from multiple personality disorder. It happens to us all. It is simply our way to make sure that we **think more holistically and balanced**. Therefore we make both rational and emotional decisions throughout our life. Most of the time, our inner mind will agree with our conscious mind and that will create a feeling of a harmonious and well-balanced life.

Here's another example. Think back at a time when you needed to make an important decision. You may have felt an inner conflict initially and then overtime, you found peace and inner contentment with the decision you made. This inner peace comes about when your inner mind is given a full opportunity to *'be heard'* and is in agreement with your more rational and analytical mind.

Your Conscious Mind	Your Subconscious (Inner) Mind
Your 'Self Talk'	*Instincts*
Your filter for all information	*Beliefs and Values*
Critical Thinking	*Habits*
Analytical Thinking	*Emotions*
Will Power	*Protective Mechanisms*
Temporary Memory	*Permanent Memory*

[6]Alman, B. & Lambrou, p., 1983, Self Hypnosis - The Complete Manual for Health and Self Change

Your conscious minds protects the inner mind

When we were children, our conscious and subconscious minds are less segregated. Children without a developed conscious mind are willing to believe what most adults tell them. They start to form values, fears and beliefs about the world and who they are, based solely on adults they are closest to. It takes many years before a child starts to have any of their 'own' beliefs.

I like the photo I found of a baby looking curiously at the tarantula spider that was crawling slowly up his arm (I didn't put the photo in here, so not to startle the arachnophobians amongst us). The baby is calm and relaxed with the spider, as he hasn't yet learnt to fear the spider as yet. If his mother and those of significance in his life don't negatively react to the spider, he will go on to warmly regard spiders or at least be indifferent to them. If his mother has a manic moment, with a blood curdling scream attached, the boy will store his mother's fear of spiders as his own inner belief, most likely for the rest of his life.

In the same way, people who have had a traumatic experience often can't fully remember the event, as our **inner mind has chosen to protect us from the experience**. So the inner mind uses protective mechanisms to shield us from our past. We often can find ourselves doing, saying or believing something that that is alarming or foreign to us.

 "An anxious mind cannot exist in a relaxed body". Edmund Jacobson

YOUR BIRTHING INNER MIND

When we come to the day our baby's birth, our inner mind with bring up all the emotions, beliefs and feelings we have about birth. We may not even know these feelings exist as our inner mind may even block our full knowledge. Yet how we feel or believe deep down is our inner mind peeping through to our lives.

For many women, they choose the Hypnobirthing Home Study Course because they want to have an amazing, natural and empowered birth. Yet on a deeper level, they just don't believe they can have that type of birth and **something is stopping them** getting to believe they will have this type of birth. These women are in conflict between what they 'want' and what they 'believe' about birth. This mismatch between 'want' and 'belief' in birthing is why we use hypnosis are a corner stone of our hypnobirthing course.

Hypnosis is a tool that allows us to change our beliefs so they are in harmony with our 'wants'. In this way, our conscious and subconscious mind is in union and this creates the inner peace and gives us the ability to truly believe in our body's ability to birth our babies in comfort and safety.

Your guard dog and your book

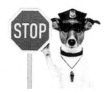 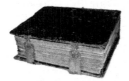

Think of your conscious mind like a guard dog, and your subconscious mind as a book of your life. In the book, you store all your life's beliefs, experiences, emotions and habits (either helpful or unhelpful). Your conscious mind will attempt to **stop thoughts that challenge** whatever you have written in your book of your life. For example, if you had a past birth where there were many negative emotions, it will be difficult for you to suddenly change your belief about birth to a more empowered view.

Your guard dog grants cautious access

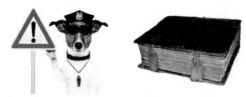

Thinking again, back to the guard dog being our conscious mind, and the book of our life is our inner mind. This time, when we are in a deeply relaxed hypnotic state, it is like the guard dog **changes the sign from 'STOP" to "Caution'**. Therefore, access to our inner mind is granted, as long as we are benefiting, not harming our subconscious mind.

When it comes to birth, the *'wanting'* to have an amazing birth is now supported by our **new belief in our ability to birth**. We find a new, fresh confidence that this birth will be the birth of our dreams. When the day of our birth finally arrives, we are naturally calm, relaxed and at peace because we know (not just hope) that we will birth easily. This is the power of hypnosis -to challenge the old inferior beliefs that we all hold about birth and install a new more positive feelings and knowingness in how we will bring a baby into the world.

> This intentional hypnosis in Hypnobirthing, is the active process of connecting into the part of the mind responsible for change. In this state, your conscious mind is not blocking suggestions, so the subconscious mind is receptive and is therefore much more likely to succeed in making the desired changes. This is far more effective than just relying on determination and willpower, which is what most people rely upon to make changes.

You are fully in control with Hypnosis

Many people are under the impression that hypnosis is something done to you when you are under someone else's control. Essentially, all hypnosis is self-hypnosis. A hypnotherapist may be able to guide you with the use of words, but then each person is completely in control of his own mind. Being so, only you can decide which suggestions and visualizations to follow. **You are in complete control** of where your mind takes you.

In the same way, if there is something that you do not agree with, then your subconscious mind WILL NOT accept or take on board the suggestions. Your inner values are stored in your subconscious mind, and if your values are against a suggestion, you will not accept it.

For example, under hypnosis, if someone directed you to rob a bank and if you hold a value that says *'robbing a bank is wrong,'* then no matter what is said under hypnosis, you will refuse to accept the direction. Therefore, you have a built in safety mechanism that only allows positive suggestions and changes of your beliefs that are helpful to you.

> Your values are stored in your subconscious mind and if your values do not support a suggestion in hypnosis, you naturally come out of the relaxed state and refuse to accept the suggestion. You are always in control.

Stage Hypnosis is still self-hypnosis

On a hypnosis stage show, there may have five people on stage and the hypnotist asks all these five to perform an act. You often will find that three of the five will happily perform the act, while two are not responsive to the suggestion. It so happens that the three who performed the act most likely would be happy to recreate this after a night out of drinking when they are in a relaxed state. On the flip side, the other two on stage refused, even when in a relaxed state. Therefore the two people on stage values systems stopped them from performing against their true desires. **Likewise, under hypnosis, you are always in control and will act only in accordance to your wishes and beliefs.**

 Mother's Thoughts

'I nearly didn't do Hypnobirthing because there was hypnosis in it. The whole thing scared me senseless. I though hypnosis was more about letting someone control your mind and get you to do weird things. I had no idea how that related to birthing anyway, it all sounded a bit strange to me. Anyway, my neighbour did hypnobirthing and she had one of the best births ever. She was chilled and just went with the flow and everything went so well. About a year before her birth, we both were terrified at even the thought of birth, crossing our legs tight at the time!

She had an amazing turnaround in what she thought about birth. She said she just now knew she could do it, and was actually looking forward to the birth! After checking her cupboards for psychotic drugs, she told me it was all down to the hypnosis in hypnobirthing. It actually changed what she believed about birth. She just was more settled and confident within herself; a changed women!

When I got pregnant, I had to give this a go. If this can make a new person out of my neighbour, then it might just work for me now as well. I am really proud to say that I had my brilliant birth as well. It was just fabulous. I became that changed women as well. Now when my neighbour and I have a chat over the fence about birth, it is all good for us'. **Victoria Archer, St Albans, England**

THE LAWS OF THE MIND

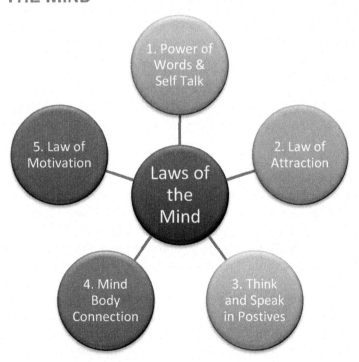

THE POWER OF WORDS AND SELF-TALK

In Hypnobirthing, the most powerful tool that is used is the spoken word. The words we say both to ourselves and others are more powerful than most people imagine.

 "Words are, of course, the most powerful drug used by mankind." Rudyard Kipling

The biggest difference between us and other animals is our ability to communicate and to use words for ourselves and with those around us. Out of words come thoughts; out of thoughts come ideas; out of ideas come inventions; and out of inventions comes "civilization". The words we use and how we use them drive our daily lives. How we think and how we speak to ourselves motivate our behaviour. In addition, the words and ideas we hear from others **create our belief systems**.

Words are the building blocks for how we live our lives. By focusing in on the words you use to yourself, you can change your entire perspective of the world: you can help heal your body, you can change your belief patterns, and you can change how you see yourself in the world.

Words motivate us for good or evil

Words spoken by a great leader can be uplifting and empowering, and can cause people to act in remarkable ways. Likewise, words spoken can create a darker community. The speeches of Hitler created a completely new mindset, a new way of thinking, a new belief system that led to some of the greatest atrocities we know today. While in the same era, the words of Winston Churchill inspired and motivated a nation.

How your parents, teachers, school friends and other significant figures in your life spoke to you will influence your actions. Their words and how they are said, would also influence how you feel about yourself for the rest of your life. The words we hear around us have enormous influence on our decisions, values and patterns of behaviour.

Whatever words we hear, we turn the interpretation of **words into an emotion.** Among these emotions would be such as fear, anger, sadness, guilt, happiness or pride. If someone criticizes you unfairly, you turn that negative feeling into energy. Likewise, if someone praises you on a great job, you turn that positive feeling into energy. All words we hear are interpreted, assigned an emotion and given energy to it. And this energy is then saved and stored in our body.

Words that we speak to ourselves

It is easy to see and feel the impact words have on us when spoken by others. Most people underestimate the strength the words they speak to themselves have on their own energy levels and energy resources.

Research shows most people have about 50,000 thoughts every day. It does sound like a lot, doesn't it? Every time one of those 50,000 thoughts takes place, chemicals are produced in your brain that can trigger reactions felt throughout your entire body. This '**Mind Body Connection**' creates a strong relationship between what you think and how you feel, both physically and emotionally. And because you are always thinking (much like breathing), you tend to forget that you are doing it. Most of the time, you don't even realise how much your thoughts dictate how you feel every minute of every single day.

It's impossible to track and monitor every single thought you have, to see if it's having a positive or negative influence on your emotional state. The thoughts that are most influential are those where you **literally talk to yourself**. Though you might not realise you have these thoughts, we all have an internal voice inside our head that affects our perception of our world. We find that we tell ourselves to keep quiet, we congratulate ourselves on an achievement, and we reprimand ourselves for making decisions we later regret. Our thoughts are "talking" to us every day, and this inner voice is called **"self-talk."**

Thoughts are the primary vehicle for regulating your emotional experience. What you allow yourself to think can rush emotions quickly to the surface, be stuffed deep down or intensify and prolong any emotional experience. When a rush of emotion comes over you, your thoughts turn the heat up or down. By learning to control yourself talk, you can keep yourself focused on the right things and manage your emotions more effectively.

Much of the time, your self-talk is neutral or even positive and it helps you through your day ("What maternity top goes with this skirt" or "I'm really looking forward to seeing the baby on the ultrasound today"). Yet, more negative self-talk is unrealistic and self-defeating. It can send you into a downward emotional spiral that makes it difficult for you to feel emotionally free and in control.

> Your thoughts are the key way to control your emotions. By learning to control your thoughts, it keeps you focused on more positive birth images and creates a happier, more balanced emotional experience.

What's your birth 'self-talk'?

The problem comes when we beat ourselves up over and over again about what we should or shouldn't do in pregnancy and birth. There is so much 'mother's guilt' floating around us when we are pregnant. We now have this enormous responsibility for bringing a baby into the world, healthy and happy. This, at times, can feel like an overwhelming burden of responsibility. Our 'baby' self-talk is often so critical that we feel that anything less than a perfect pregnancy, birth and baby would make us less of a mother.

I spoke to one new mother who had given birth naturally using hypnobirthing. I thought it was a beautiful 'text book' Hypnobirth. It was a relatively short and easy labor with the 'chilled out' baby girl delivered free of intervention. So I would have thought this new mother would be over the moon with joy. Wrong! This mother went on to list all the things that didn't go right on the day.

- I visualized my labor would be less than five hours and it was nine hours!
- My husband forgot how to use the relaxation trigger and he messed up the massage!
- I was expecting no pain at all and I was really annoyed that at I felt some pain at transition for about thirty minutes.
- The midwife asked me about my pain levels once, when I specifically had it written on the birth plan, no questions about pain!

This mother later went on to say to me, '*I wanted my birth to be perfect. It is not a true Hypnobirth unless it is perfect!*' Most of us would think that she overreacted to the more minor details of her birth and lost sight of the bigger picture. I would say that is a fair assessment, yet it is easy to cling so tight to a **view of perfection** that we miss out on the joy of life that is right here in our hands. We often let the smallest detail suffocate the beautiful breathing and vibrant picture.

Quick Exercise: How will you be at your birth? Will you focus on the few negatives and be oblivious to the wonderful, exciting and amazing birth adventure? As you give this some real thought, take a look closer to home and think back over your own pregnancy so far. What has been your self-talk? Have you reacted to things that aren't that important?

With any significant event in our life like birth, we have so much vested interested in getting everything just perfect. In the process, we just forget to *enjoy* our pregnancy and birth. Have you ever seen a 'Bridezilla?' I never, ever thought I would become one. Yet, at my own wedding, I hit the roof when I noticed the caterers opened two bottles of expensive champagne close to the end of the night, and then poured them down the sink ten minutes later. Whether it is your wedding, an important event, or pregnancy and birth, remember most of all: **really enjoy each and every day.** Give yourself a break from being perfect, as nothing will ever be perfect, no matter how tight you hold onto your ideals.

Three tips for controlling negative self-talk

If you start to follow these suggestions, you will find that in a very short space of time, you have significantly reduced your negative self-talk. You are now brimming with a more positive outlook that will benefit not only you, but your baby as well. Any feelings no matter what form they take are transferred directly to your baby. **Your baby is a magnet for your emotional mood.** One of the most important things you can do to grow a healthy baby is to think and feel positive and uplifting thoughts.

Here's how to take control of your emotional well-being: **1. Swap, 2. Replace and 3. Accept.**

1. Swap - '*I always* or *I never*' with -'*just this time* or *sometimes*'.
Your actions are unique to the situation in front of you, no matter how often you think you messed up. Make certain your thoughts follow suit. Don't beat yourself up - it's just not helpful. When you start treating each situation as on its own and stop criticizing yourself up over every mistake, you'll stop making your problems bigger than they really are. You will also find that you naturally are more receptive for change next time.

Swap – 'I always forget to take my pregnancy vitamins' **with** 'I forgot to take my pregnancy vitamins this time'.
Swap – 'I'll never grow a healthy baby; I ate so much junk today' **with** 'I ate so much junk today, but I know it's just one day and won't have any real effect on the health of my baby'.

2. Replace judgments - '*I'm an idiot*' with facts - '*I made an error*'.
Thoughts that attach a permanent label to you feel as if they are final and you can never change. Factual statements are more objective, situational and help you to focus on what you can change.

Replace – 'I am such an idiot for forgetting my doctor's appointment' **with** 'I made a mistake, I forgot my doctor's appointment this time. How can I remember for next time?'
Replace – 'I am such a klutz buying the wrong size baby clothes' **with** 'So, I got it wrong and didn't read the label this time. It happens.'

3. Accept responsibility for only your own actions.
The blame game and negative self-talk go hand in hand. If you are someone who often thinks either *it's my entire fault or it's their entire fault,* you are wrong most the time. It's commendable to accept responsibility for your actions, but not when you carry someone else's burden. Likewise, if you're always blaming others, it's time to take responsibility for your part.

If you are hounded by negative self-talk, remember to keep this under control for the sake of your own well-being and that of your baby. This new life skill will allow you to learn to quickly fix your mistakes, grow as an individual, and become more self-aware. The more you develop this now, just think how strong your skills will be when it comes time to teaching your children. What a solid, positive, and self-assured role model you will become!

If you think you are beaten, you are.
If you think you dare not, you don't.
If you'd like to win, but think you can't,
It's almost certain you won't.
If you think you'll lose, you've lost.
For out of the world we find
Success begins with a person's will.
It's all in the state of mind.
If you think you're outclassed, you are.
You've got to think high to rise.
You've got to be sure of yourself before
You can ever win a prize.
Life's battles don't always go
To the stronger or faster person.
But sooner or later the person who wins
Is the one who thinks they can. **Anonymous**

THE LAW OF ATTRACTION

The book and movie 'The Secret' by Rhonda Byrne concisely explains the law of attraction. It's been sweeping the world over the past few years, with a profound impact on people's lives. The Law of Attraction, in simple terms states;

'When you think a thought you are also attracting like thoughts to you. Whether they are good thoughts or bad thoughts, it makes no difference. And your current thoughts are creating your future life. What you think about the most or focus on the most will appear as your life.'[7]

Henry Ford said, *'If you think you can or think you can't, you're right'*. Others may know the law of attraction as simple quotes of *'Positive things happen to positive people'*. Or *'The thing I feared the most, happened to me'*. You are getting what you feeling and thinking about; that's why so many people tend to spiral into a bad day. If they trip over something getting out of bed, often their entire day seems to go like that. We strangely tend to look at days as a whole; *'I had a bad day'* or *'I had a good day'*. Rather than just saying *'the first twenty seconds when I tripped over weren't great, but the rest of the day was superb.'* It tends to be *'I had a bad day; it was just like one thing after the other went wrong'*.

What can you do?

Just shifting your emotions can change your entire day. If you start out having a good day and you're in that particular happy feeling, as long as you don't allow something to change your mood, you're going to continue to attract, more situations, and people and that sustain that happy feeling. That's just the law of attraction and how it works.

We all know people who are positive, happy and focused on what they want, and it seems life just smile upon them constantly. We also know others who are more somber and negative in their outlook on life. They are the ones who seem to be magnets for bad luck, unable to get out of the cloud that is hanging over them.

I remember my dad once said; *'Out of the four grown up children we have, two just sail through life and seem to get anything they want. It's just uncanny how things turn around for them. I guess they*

---

[7]Byrne, Rhonda. 'The Secret': Simon & Schuster Ltd, 2006

are lucky. And the other two children really struggle. It's one problem after another. We tend to have it as a standing joke, asking what went wrong this time!'

It should be no surprise that the two children, my dad was describing as 'lucky' have always been more positive people, even from a young age. The other two children, who appear to be a magnet for 'bad luck,' would have been classed as more negative in their outlook from childhood. Then my dad spoke of me out of the four children. Was he categorizing me as 'lucky' or 'unlucky'? Well, actually, I was the 'unlucky' one. And I fully agreed with him.

Fortunately, that conversation was ten years ago, and since that time, I can say that my parents have four 'lucky' children. After reading about the law of attraction, I decided to apply its lessons to my life and the results are amazing. I had to work hard at keeping my negative self-talk under control and monitor my thoughts for daydreaming about worst case scenarios (something I did often!). Am I blessed to be a naturally positive person? No, not at all! But just like you can, I can decided to live a different life. We can choose to focus on the positive aspects of life and believe for a better future for us and our family.

The law of attraction and birthing?

As you travel through your hypnobirthing journey, set your mind on a **positive experience** right from the start. You can do this by using only positive words, thoughts and phrases when describing pregnancy and birth. This will go a long way to staying in your **bubble of peace** and feel protected. Let the words that others use bounce right off it.

By staying so positive, you won't even allow the words of all those 'well meaning' friends and strangers to pass their own birth experiences to you. Remember, this is *your* birth and *your* experience, not theirs. Remind yourself that your way of thinking about birth is changing for the better and you need to reinforce this every day with thoughts, words and beliefs that are positive.

Do you constantly worry about having a painful birth with intervention or create images and scenarios in your mind where everything goes wrong with your birth? The fear of the unknown causes most of us to run these scenarios again and again in our mind.

According to the law of attraction;

1. If you **think** these thoughts,
2. **Feel** these emotions and
3. **Visualize** these outcomes;

    …then that is what is being attracted to you. It's as we have said in our minds *'we really want to have a long painful disappointing births'.*

Are you hypnotizing yourself with bad birth outcomes?

Just like we use positive thinking, hypnosis and visualization in hypnobirthing, to create amazing birth experiences, it is equally possible to use these tools to create a birth that is full of intervention, fear and disappointment.

If you are in your 'own world,' daydreaming about a more negative birth outcome, you have entered into a *natural hypnotic state* and thoughts are now bypassing your critical mind and **entering directly into your inner mind**. You are now **self-hypnotized**! These fearful thoughts are now *forming your beliefs and values* about what you really expect your birth to become.

In addition, you are using the powerful tool of visualization and visualising a bad birth outcome. As you are still in this hypnotic state, your visualizations have more power to create your future. You are unknowingly instructing your mind that this is the birth outcome you wish to have. Your inner mind stores this information as your 'desire' and 'plan' for your birth. Your inner mind or subconscious mind doesn't pass judgment on what is a positive or negative. It assumes that if you are thinking, feeling and visualizing something then that is what you 'want' to happen, even if you don't.

If you are **thinking** 'I really don't want to be induced'.

If you are **feeling** disappointment and sadness.

If you are **visualizing** being induced.

Then you have stored the plan as what you '*want*' to happen for your birth. Your inner mind now has this information and thinks you want this to happen. As your mind and body are interconnected, your mind *may* send a message to your body to start to create a situation where you can be induced, and feel disappointment and sadness.

Oh no! I thought a bad birth thought!

Now did you pick up on the word '*may*' send a message to your body? That means, if you just happen to find yourself in the induction thinking, feeling and visualising scenario above, it doesn't mean that you will automatically have an induction; nor does it mean that this is a new belief.

Think of the formation of our **beliefs as a set of scales**. You will notice there is a **tipping point** as to what will create a new belief. So you need to think, feel and visualize a lot of negatives to actually do any damage.

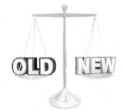

Think about your views on birth before starting the hypnobirthing course. I bet they were formed by years and years of input from family, friends, TV or movies, books, and etc. that when all combined formed your beliefs on what type of birth you will have. Perhaps your birth belief scale is already tipped into old, less helpful thinking patterns.

I recently saw a program where tribal aboriginal women of Australia spoke about 'birthing in the bush.' They fully embraced birth and the aboriginal women were fortunate to come from a culture that believed birth to be intuitive, natural and empowering. These pregnant women's thoughts and the thoughts of the entire tribe supported this natural, easy and safe birth view. It would be no surprise, really. With such a strong positive communal mindset that these tribal midwives continually got the results they expected – good birth outcomes.

> When you think of the formation of a new belief as a set of scales, the tipping point is 51%, so you will need to be thinking negatively about your birth more than good thoughts, to make any lasting changes.

Interrupt and replace negative birth scenarios

Where are your thoughts, feelings and daydreams? Are they continually focused on having the calm fulfilling birth that so many women around the world actually have? If you don't want a disappointing birth scenario to happen in your birthing, find a way to **interrupt that thought and replace with another positive one**.

For me, when I was pregnant with my twins and I happened to find myself daydreaming about getting a complication, I would mentally replay the **'uup –ummm sound'** which was like the button you hear on those game shows. Then I would visualize a healthy, happy situation in my head. It made a great deal of difference monitoring my thoughts and feelings. I felt as if I had wiped clean that scenario from my mind, just like a kid's Etch-A-Sketch, it was gone forever. By replacing the scenario with a more positive one, it gave me a quick way to feel empowered and refocused on my birth that **I really want**.

So next time, if you find yourself thinking, feeling, or visualising a less than perfect birth, **'uup – ummm' it!** And stop the thought right on its tracks. Then quickly either visualize a better birth outcome or feel more positive feelings and thoughts. In no time at all, you will find yourself thinking negatively much less often and the best benefit is; you will feel wonderful, happy and content and start think of yourself, as a positive person.

Did I cause my past bad birth outcome?

No, fundamentally not! You are not responsible for everything in life. You are not responsible for the actions of the doctors, midwives or the birthing place. You are not responsible for the actions of others, or circumstances out of your control.

In birth, like other aspects in life, things just happen and we can't do anything about them. Life happens and we are just one small part of this vast universe. We are no more responsible for a birth complication, than we are responsible for the floods, droughts or environmental disasters. So it is important not to blame yourself for outcomes, either in birth or throughout your life.

> *Some people think that if they followed the Law of Attraction correctly, then they can only have a perfect birth outcome. While the Law of Attraction is a powerful law of the mind, and is what many people have credited for their wonderful births; it is just one piece of the puzzle. We can only be responsible for ourselves and can't control others and circumstances.*

If you feel that with the new knowledge of hypnobirthing you would make different choices this time around, well, that is what this course is all about! Even if you did feel your choices in the past contributed to (not caused) a less than positive birth experience, please don't blame yourself. Remember the devastation effect that 'self-talk' can have on our minds, and this emotion is passed directly to your baby.

> **Replace** 'I am responsible for my past birth outcome' **with** 'I only had a part to play in the outcome, and I'm learning new ways to have a good birth outcome this time'.

We can be the most positive person in the world, know all the Hypnobirthing techniques and still have a complication that changes the course of our birth. Unfortunately, that is just how it can go, no matter how much we want things to go differently. The empowering part of Hypnobirthing is it gives you the tools to make effective decisions regarding the path of your birth. So you will feel in control and ready for whatever turn life takes you.

THINK AND SPEAK POSITIVELY

I remember the time when my twins were eighteen months of age and they had just pulled some leaves off a tree. They were just gazing down at the leaves in their own little word, pleased with their new ability to yank the leaves off the branches all by themselves. My husband then said, *'Don't put the leaves in your mouth.'* At once and in unison, the twins placed the leaves in their mouths and started to chew on them. It was if they had heard the command *'put the leaves in your mouth'* and completely disregarded the *'don't'*. I'm sure I could see the clogs turning in their minds. *'Oh, what a good idea! I hadn't thought about putting the leaves in my mouth before.'*

If you have a toddler, you will understand when I say that young children have trouble understanding and following through on a *'negative' request*. These would be; 'Don't, Not', No, Shouldn't, Wouldn't, etc'.

Don't eat the dirt.

No hurting the cat.

That's **not** good for you.

Young children are more likely to comply with a *'positive' request*; one where the request is clearer to them. Here are a few examples:

Eating dirt will make you sick. Here, the grapes are better to eat.

Stop. That's making the cat sore.

That's yucky, this is nicer.

If you can **reduce** the 'Don't, No and Not' in your language, it is found that children will learn much faster what is acceptable and inappropriate behaviour.

Adult's minds and 'negatives'

We know to limit the negatives when we are around young children. But how does that affect us as adults now? Surely, we can easily process the 'Don't, No and Not', Shouldn't and Wouldn't?

Quick Exercise: Try this little test: *Whatever you do, **don't** think of a blue castle.*

In order you to **not** think of a blue castle; you actually had to create a blue castle in your mind first. Therefore, initially your mind has the **same response** to '***Don't*** *think of a blue castle and* '***think*** *of a blue castle.*

The same is true for *'don't, not and no'* and anything that we have that creates a negative for us. The minute you say *'don't'* the inner mind deletes that word and actually does the opposite; therefore, the **words need to be positive when instructing your inner mind.** Sound strange? Ok, try this one:

Quick Exercise: *You know the moon is **not** made out of green cheese, so **do not** think of green cheese.* Did you see in your mind, even for a moment, green cheese?

I mentioned that our *inner mind* has trouble understanding a negative and works in positives by deleting the negative word. Yet, you may have noticed that when you did the blue castle and green cheese example, your inner mind created the image for you for **only a moment**. And then your *critical mind*, being the more logical and analytic, interoperated what was actually being said and removed the imaged. Therefore, your critical mind, can understand the 'don't, not, no, never, needn't, haven't etc' and easily follow through on a 'negative request'.

'Don't clean up the mess, I'd do it later'.

'No, I don't like that tie'.

'Never, eat that, it makes you bloated'.

Your critical mind can clearly interpret a 'negative'; yet your inner mind deletes a 'negative'. In hypnosis, we have greater access to our inner mind, so we need to use more positive words and phrases.

Back to toddlers minds again

The reason why toddlers need to be directed in clear, positive terms is due to the fact that their inner and critical minds are less separated. Young children operate mainly from their inner minds and initially only respond with their inner minds, so the 'negative' is deleted straight away. *'Don't put the dirt in your mouth*, becomes a command of *'put the dirt in your mouth'*. The toddler's inner mind is more instinctive and quick to react to the command and sure enough, the dirt is in the mouth. Then the less developed critical mind in the toddler may have caught up with understanding what the *'don't'* actually means and then spat the dirt out. (I am sure the taste would also be a prompt!).

If you don't have your own toddler, go the park and see if you can observe one for a bit and notice the almost dazed, hypnotic state that these kids find themselves in most of the time. That is their inner mind being most present. You may even notice that some parents are becoming more and more frustrated with their toddlers behaviour and the tension building with '**No! Don't'** eat the dirt. **Haven't** I told you so many times?' The poor parents are frazzled and the toddler looks confused.

Negatives and Hypnobirthing

As we are more readily accessing our *inner mind in hypnobirthing* in the same way toddlers automatically do, we focus on using positive phrases and suggestions during your birthing.

For example, birth partners: instead of saying things like '***Don't*** *tense up'* why not say; *'Now relax that part of your body.'* So you are always directing your inner mind what to do and we do that by speaking in only positive terms when we are in a hypnotic state.

Is your self-talk full of negatives? Do you find yourself daydreaming in a self-hypnotic state, while feeling the emotion and saying to yourself: 'I **don't** want a caesarean,' 'I'll **never** need an epidural,' and I'm **not** having intervention'. All of these phrases makes us think, feel and focus our attention on the actual things we don't want. If you say these with emotions, you are accessing your inner mind when and leaving an instruction for:

> I want a caesarean.
>
> I'll need an epidural.
>
> I'm having intervention.

Is one or even a few thoughts going to make that much difference? No, remember the scales in our self-talk section? For any thought, we must be thinking it, feeling it and visualising it **more than half the time to have a lasting effect and install a belief**.

Relax! A stray thought here and there will not do undo the good work that you have done to create a wonderful birth for yourself. On the flip side of that equation, we must be thinking more positive thoughts, feelings and visualizations.

So that is why positive thoughts, messages, affirmations, watching great births and listening to our hypnobirthing class recordings will constantly remind us of what we *actually do what*. We think positive thoughts, feel great about our birthing and change our thinking when it is not in line with what we actually want.

How does the hypnosis side of hypnobirthing relate to birthing? In short, hypnosis makes it easier for us to make the changes in our thought and feelings. In all Hypnobirthing Home Study Course recordings, we focus on positive language and encourage you to create your own amazing birth story in your mind. The more you run these types of images through your mind and actually feel and experience your best birth experiences, your mind and body respond to create your perfect birth.

In hypnosis, you deeply relax and just give yourself permission to accept the positive birthing suggestions. By being deeply relaxed, you allow yourself to travel past the critical and logical part of your mind so the messages can go into your inner mind or subconscious mind, and make real and lasting change. **The more you listen to the Hypnobirthing Home Study Course recordings, you will find you are naturally being more positive about your birth**, believe you can and will have a fulfilling and easy birth. In time, there won't even be any negative thoughts to monitor.

Your self-talk will be positive, the changes so natural, easy and effective. You would have changed your thinking to what it should have been in the first place; that birth is natural, wonderful, empowering and intuitive. And as a woman, you have this right to have this amazing birth experience.

Hypnobirthing words are positive and uplifting

The words we use create thoughts and emotions; repeatedly entertaining the same thoughts conjures up feelings. In time, these feelings become our beliefs. Once those beliefs are established, we automatically begin to act out those beliefs with our behaviour. Positive behaviours create positive experiences; negative behaviours create negative experiences. Therefore, in hypnobirthing, we focus only on the positive.

Hypnobirthing parents learn to use language that describes what is happening within the birthing mother's body during birth. This more gentle language is found to be meaningful to parents than language that is medicalised.

The language you use and the language you hear from people around you, should keep your mind in a state of calm and keep away from triggering a state of stress and fear. Learn to choose your words carefully. **Associate with people where you can, who reinforce your own positive thinking** about birthing. If you are being hounded by people who want to tell you disappointing birth stories, suggest that you wait until after you have your baby's birth to exchange tales of birth. Say '*I've made a decision not to hear other people's birth stories, until after the birth. Perhaps we can talk then*'. This will be a quick, easy and non-judgmental way of stopping a birth negativity seeping through.

When you have this positive thinking, speaking and living, as well as the support from your partner, friends and family; this will help you to work together toward a the most positive birth experience. This calmness and focus will be automatically there for you during birthing, and spill over into every aspect of your life.

To truly embrace the concept of gentle, natural and normal birth, learn to think and speak in the kinder, softer word. Once you start to think in more positive birth terms, it will be easier to believe in the birth you are truly after. That said, you will find that most doctors and midwives will ask about your contraction, talk about the fetus and discuss your labor. While it is important to think in more positive terms, we cannot force the whole medical establishment to change their language, and so it is necessary remove any strong associations with the more medical words. That is why, throughout the Hypnobirthing Home Study Course, we mostly use the softer hypnobirthing language and importantly sprinkle in the medicalised language as well. In this way, you can have a more positive response to both language styles and relax at your birth.

Medicalised Language	Hypnobirthing Language
Pain	Discomfort
Contractions	Surge, pressure, sensations, tightening

Labor	Your birthing time
Fetus	Your baby
Water Breaking	Membranes Releasing
Deliver the baby	Birthing your baby
Due Date	Birth Guestimate
Birth Coach	Birth Partner
Pushing	Birth Breathing
Complications	Change of Plans
Birth Canal	Birth Path
Bloody Show	Birth Show
Effacing/Dilating	Thinning and Opening
False Labor	Practice Labor
Active Labor	Established Birthing

 It's essential that you keep your thoughts and language focused on what you do want rather than creating wasted negative energy around circumstances that you don't want. Tune into only positive thoughts, feelings and language and feel the difference in your emotions.

Mother's Thoughts

"I very much wanted a great birth, but I felt such a constant struggle between what I really wanted and what I thought would have to happen. I had this belief deep down that no matter what I thought or did, I still would end up with the same result, a long and painful birth. My fate was sealed; I couldn't do anything about it. There was this constant nagging in the back of my mind. Sometimes I felt it was a bit of a lost cause doing the Hypnobirthing Home Study Course, as in the early days of study, I would read one of the Mother's thoughts and feel great about my birth and then start to think, I may actually be one of those women who have fantastic births. Yet, it was like I had this gremlin, taking control of my mind again and tell me that my birth will be nothing like theirs; it will be just horrible and painful.

I continued with the course and I am so glad I did! It made all the difference, I worked on my self-talk and often it felt as if I was forcing myself to be positive, like a battle raging in my mind. Yet with all the self-talk tips and the help of the releasing fears CD, I won the war! Yeah!!

I was quite surprised how fast it took; within a week I felt I had completely changed my thought process. I went through a whole day and by the end of it, I realised that I didn't have any bad thoughts at all about birth; just a whole lot of good positive vibes flowing in. The best thing is, I was happier now than I have ever been.

I am so proud and happy to say, that I gave birth to my beautiful baby girl, Amelia on 6.03am on Sunday morning. The birth was just like my visualization (the good ones). I can't wait to tell everyone about the Hypnobirthing Home Study Course, it made my birth the best experience of my life. Thanks so much for your help. I know without the course, I would have let that gremlin win for sure". **Olivia White, Waiheke Island, New Zealand**

THE MIND BODY CONNECTION

Every thought causes a physical reaction.

Quick Exercise: Really think about a mortifying experience from your past, (I'm sure there are many for all of us) and just notice how your body reacts to just the memory of the experience. Give it a moment to recall the experience and feel what it is to be there right now.

What has changed in your body from recalling the memory?

For every suggestion, thought or emotion one entertains, there is a corresponding physiological and chemical response within the body. Dr. Al Krazner, 'The Wizard Within'.

Your mind is a General: your body a Soldier

Our bodies obey the instructions of our minds. Think of our mind as a General giving commands and our body as an obedient soldier who carries out an order without question or judgment. What is experienced in the body is determined in the mind. Therefore, what the mind chooses to accept or perceive as being real, the soldier body, accordingly responds to the command. The mind does not have the ability to act, so it sends messages to the body demanding action. The body, in turn, plays out the thought.

Cast your minds back to high school science and remember Pavlov's experiment with dogs. The dogs over time became conditioned to salivate in anticipation of receiving food at the ringing of a bell. This perhaps the most commonly recognised example of a mind-body connection.

We experience this law every day of our lives. The sight of a police car on the road automatically slows our driving, no matter what our speed. The red traffic light conditions us to stop. The sirens of an ambulance make us instantly jump to attention. An unexpected object on our path startles us and we may involuntarily cry out or gasp. If there is an unexpected person lurking in the shadows, the mind - body reaction is even stronger. As your mind registers danger approaching, your body responds by preparing for the situation. The anxiety and fear create a surge of adrenaline which increases your pulse rate, breathing and direct blood to your arms and legs (flight or fight response) and shuts down non-essential processes such as digestion.

Created emotions have the same effect as real emotions

I can't even watch a horror movie at night and I had to ban myself from watching them. I know the horror is not real, but I just keep getting drawn into the movie and then I find myself lying wide awake at night, pumped up with adrenaline, with no hope of getting to sleep. Do I really think it is logical for an axe-wielding alien with two heads and dripping orange ooze to attack me in my bed tonight? Not entirely likely. Yet my mind still 'believes' this will happen on some level. So my body responds to my mind accordingly and continues to send through the surge of adrenaline and keep me awake and grant me the best chance of survival. With the adrenaline pumping, I can either fight off the alien attack or run for my life. It is only when I am more rational again and *changed my thinking* to that of calm relaxing thoughts. My body can calm again and stop sending 'survival' messages to my body. Yet, for the next day, I find myself on edge just a little.

I am sure there you many other examples in your own life. Perhaps where you thought or daydreamed about something that wasn't actually true and noticed your body's stress reaction over the situation. I remember one mother say to me that she has a habit of letting her imagination run away with her and this time she *imagined* her husband forgot her birthday, which was over a month away. She felt her blood increase and felt so angry and hostile with him for this supposed crime he had committed. Then she dismissed this thought as nonsense after a few minutes. Later on, she couldn't work out why she was so angry and aloof to her husband when he came home that night. She seemed eager to start a fight and let off some steam.

The next time you find yourself experiencing an emotion or reaction in your body that seems to just appear, stop for a moment and ask yourself, *'Is this due to something that I thought, felt or daydreamed about?'*

THE INNER WORKING OF THE UTERUS

To fully understand the effect of the mind-body connection on birthing, we must first look at the role the uterus in our birthing time. So please take a quick anatomy lesson with me.

Hypnobirthing simplifies the uterine layers into two sections

1. The outer **longitudinal muscle** fibers (aligned up and down with your body).

  During a surge, these muscles tighten and draw up the (relaxed) circular muscles at the neck of the uterus; they cause the edges of the cervix to progressively thin and open.

  In an almost wave like motion, these long muscles shorten and flex to nudge the baby down, through and ultimately out of the uterus.

2. The inner **circular muscle** layers found mostly at the lower part of the uterus (surrounding your baby). In order for the uterus to open and allow the baby to move easily down, through and out of the uterus into the birth canal, these lower, thicker muscles have to relax and thin.

Your normal birthing uterus

In a normal, natural birthing situation, a mother is fully relaxed and trusts her body to birth her baby effectively. She trusts that her birthing muscles know what to do when the time is right. She knows her muscles are working perfectly together to thin, soften and open her cervix, ready for her baby to pass through her open uterus and then down the birth path to meet her.

For every surge, she practices surge breathing, which has such a calming effect on her body and mind. This deep relaxation allows her body and her uterine muscles to work in harmony with each other, easily and effectively. Each time she feels the warmth and power of a surge, her longitudinal muscles tighten and this tightening draws up the relaxed and passive circular muscles. This pulling up of the non-resistant circular muscles allows the edges of the cervix to gradually thin and open. **As long as the circular muscles stay passive, relaxed and compliant to the tightening and pulling up of the longitudinal muscles, then all is going well with birthing**. This almost wave like motion of the muscles working together, creates a feeling of comfort in the birthing mother. She reports only the feeling the tightness and then release of the surge. As long as the circular muscles stay relaxed and passive, the longitudinal muscles are free to nudge the baby down and ultimately out of the uterus.

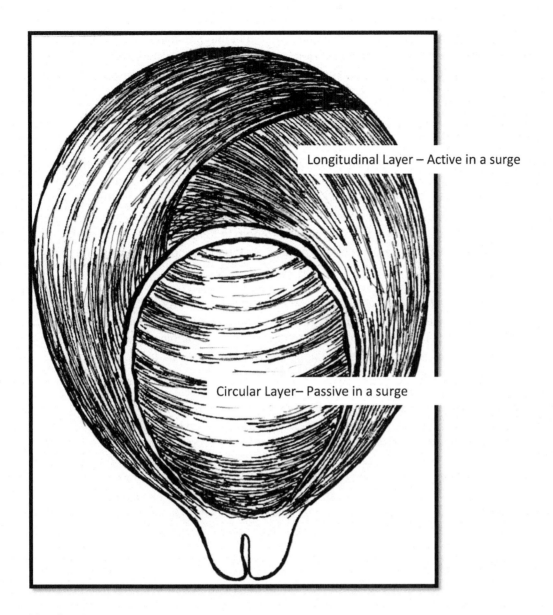

Longitudinal Layer – Active in a surge

Circular Layer– Passive in a surge

Uterine Layers

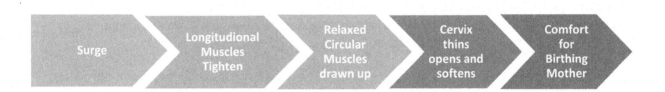

Surge → Longitudional Muscles Tighten → Relaxed Circular Muscles drawn up → Cervix thins opens and softens → Comfort for Birthing Mother

The normal, natural surge

Fear affects your surges

The uterus muscles are beautifully designed to deal quite effectively with danger, fear and stress in your birthing time. The uterus is the only muscle in the body that contains within itself two opposing muscle groups, one to induce and continue labor (the longitudinal muscles) and another to stop labor if the birthing mother is in danger or is afraid (contraction of the usually passive circular muscles).

Emotional or physical stress will automatically signal danger to a birthing mammal and her labor will slow down or stop completely so that she can move quickly to safety. It makes sense that nature designed our body so that we can stop or slow labor if a wild animal is lurking in our village and start up labor again once the threat has gone.

Our thoughts and emotions can slow or stop labor

In modern times, we tend not to have too many physical threats to stop labor, but we know that our thoughts and emotions control our bodily responses. And as our mind doesn't readily distinguish between real and imagined fears, it will send the same message of adrenaline rushing through our veins to ensure the best possible chance of survival. This surge of adrenaline will normally give us the ability to run faster than we have before or find new found strength to fight off an attack. In some cases, people have harnessed the power of adrenaline with new found strength to lift cars and drag loved ones to safety.

Yet in birthing situation, we *can't run* from our fears, which may include a horror birthing story from our best friend, what we saw on TV as a child, the hospital environment, or something the midwife said. We *can't fight* either. Well, this is not the readily accepted behaviour in a birthing situation, although women in birthing have been known scream, attack and verbally abuse their partners. (That is, the non-hypnobirthing mothers of cause!)

Instead, if there are thoughts of fear or anxiety, our body responds like any other situation where our minds feel threatened. It's as if our mind has actually said to our body, *"… I understand it is not 'safe' to give birth now, so I will release adrenaline to stop or slow down the progression of labor.'* The only way your mind knows you are safe, and everything is OK, is by your thoughts and feelings. When you are relaxed, calm again, thinking good thoughts and feeling positive, then and only then, does your mind perceive the *'threat to labor'* is gone. As your mind returns to a more positive state, then your mind instructs your body that all is well again and requests the flow of adrenaline to stop. At this time, with the adrenaline out of your body, labor can start again or resume more effectively.

Adrenaline causes the uterus to 'fight' labor

Remember back to a uterus section? Only the longitudinal muscles are contracting. The circular muscles are passive and allow the longitudinal muscles to draw then up and open, thin and soften the cervix. Yet, the rush of **adrenaline causes the short circular muscle fibers of the lower uterus to contract.** The contractions of these circular muscles are responsible for stopping or slowing labor by closing and tightening the cervix. At the same time the long, straight **longitudinal muscle fibers of the uterus are keeping on doing what is required,** so they continue to contract in an attempt to prepare your cervix for birth. The short circular muscles of the lower uterus are also contracting to keep the cervix closed and 'flight' the labor.

What is the result of this 'fight'? The very real pain of **two powerful muscles pulling in opposite directions** each time the birthing mother has a contraction. No longer are the muscles working in harmony, flowing rhythmically with each surge, they are now at war with each other, both **contracting with opposite agendas.** These conflicting messages within the body will cause pain and complications.

Adrenaline creates pain for you and your baby

With the cervix closed tight, with each contraction, the longitudinal muscles push the baby's head against taut muscles, and this additional pressure can cause **pain for both baby and mother.** The weight of the baby's head on a tighten cervix while being pushed down continually causes discomfort for the mother. After all, the cervix is not designed to take that weight. A mother won't like the experience of this extra pressure, and the baby doesn't either, as the baby is being squashed with each contraction, but has nowhere to go.

In addition, with both muscles contracting means there is **limited oxygen to the uterus**, also means the supply to the baby is compromised. So, over a period of time, this can be a cause for concern. The baby is often classified as **'in distress.'** In addition, the mother is not dilating or progressing in her labor and the situation is often called **'failure to progress'**, and usually results in **intervention.**[8]

Adrenaline neutralizes hormones

When a woman has adrenaline in her system during birth, she will have extreme discomfort due to the uterus muscles are in **conflict with each other**. In addition, the adrenalin neutralizes the wonderful birthing hormones, including oxytocin (the one that makes the uterus contract and release), endorphins (natural painkillers) and relaxin (helps with elasticity of the muscles). The hormones, oxytocin and endorphins influence the degree to which we interpret feelings as pain or pleasure. **If you reduce these hormones, then the perception of pain will significantly increase.**

FEAR-TENSION-PAIN

"The strain in pain lies mainly in the brain."
The fear-tension-pain phrase was first coined by Grantly Dick-Read in 1942[9], following his study of women who gave birth and did not feel significant pain. **Fear results in tension; tension results in pain; pain leads to fear of the next contraction and the cycle is repeated.** Dick-Read believed that birth is not naturally painful and that it was culturally induced fears that played a significant part in the pain cycle. All of these factors have the ability to slow down or even stop labor, and a woman going through this truly does experience severe pain, which in turn reinforces the fear of the next contraction, and so the cycle goes on.

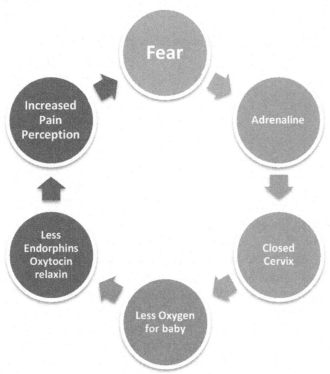

---

[8]Lederman, R. P. etal., "Anxiety and epinephrine in multiparous women in labor: relationship to duration of labor and fetal heart rate pattern". Am J Obstet Gynecol 1985;153(8):870-7.

[9]Dick-Read, G.,2004, Childbirth without Fear, page 45; Pinter & Martin Ltd.

Fear-Tension- Pain causes intervention

As you can see, a woman can become so entrenched in this horrible cycle that her body continues to hold back from birthing her baby. This may partly explain the current drastically high rates of chemical augmentation of labor and **increase of Caesarean sections due to "failure to progress."** This is the most common reason for unplanned Caesarean sections today. The fear-tension-pain may also help to explain the rising rate of inductions as the fear of birth may even prevent some women going into spontaneous labor.

> If a woman says her birth was painful, perhaps it was because of the rush of adrenaline creating this cycle of fear. Remember, with Hypnobirthing you will be so relaxed and calm, you will flow with the natural, normal and comfortable way of birthing.

What happens to a non-Hypnobirthing mother-to-be?

In a hospital environment where a non-hypnobirthing mother-to-be is scared about birth and the contractions have stopped or slowed down; one of the treatment options is to give the mother an epidural. In this way, the mother can get some sleep, have time to relax and realise that she is in fact OK and so is her baby. With the adrenaline now out of her system, like a charm, labor contractions often reappear and progress is now made.

Also, it is quite common for labors to go well, and having comfortable surges with good dilation occurring, in a home situation. Then when women appear in the hospital environment and overcome with medical equipment, comments from the medical staff, sounds from other birthing women, that it all becomes too much and now the previously calm and well progressed labor suddenly starts to become painful and progression has slowed and intervention offered.

Clearing your fears is such an important part of having calm and fulfilling birth and we will be doing that later in this unit.

> Being relaxed in your birthing time, results in relaxed muscles with no resistance, low adrenaline levels, helpful hormones and plenty of oxygen to your muscles and to baby, so you feel calm and comfortable.

Using the mind-body connection for your amazing birth

Utilizing this law so that it works with and for you during your birthing is essential. We know that if the focus of birth is on fearful, negative images, the body is thrown unintentionally into a defense mode. The physical response then becomes the enemy to normal birthing function.

As you go through this course, you will become skilled in using your own natural abilities to bring your **mind and body into psycho-physical harmony**. The thoughts you use and practice are those that will condition your body and your mind to create endorphins (neuropeptides that create a feeling of wellbeing). You will also learn special deepening techniques that will help you to connect with your baby and work with your body to bring yourself even deeper level of relaxation and comfort as your labor progresses.

THE LAW OF MOTIVATION

What you want is what you get

You can't help but be accosted by everyone you meet when you are pregnant. It seems you now have a sign across your belly: 'Please tell me your birthing horror story; the more gruesome the details the better'. It is almost as though people think it is their solemn duty as citizens to inform you of traumatic births, an education of sort. They assume you are naïve, uneducated, or ill-informed about birth. As such, you will appreciate their insightful stories and thank them wholeheartedly for their education!

Well, as crazy as it sounds, we are as primed to be drawn to wanting to listen to these sensationalized stories! Traumatic birth stories are no exception. I was surprised to hear that in my own mother's group. Out of the six mothers, two of us had natural easy births through hypnobirthing, two had minor interventions with manageable pain, and two had difficult births. When we got together to discuss our births, it was interesting to note the interaction and dynamics in the group. The two of us who had easy natural births openly discussed our births. There was no acknowledgment that we put a lot of effort to train our minds and body to have a great birth. *'Oh you got it easy'* and *'I'm sure you just have a high pain threshold'*. Interestingly we actually started feeling apologetic for having great fulfilling births, crazy as it seems.

We were abruptly interrupted by the ones who had the difficult birth. It seems easy births are *'too boring'* for the group and the Shakespearian dramatics of the difficult births were played out in minute detail. As I looked around the room, it became clear that everyone was on the edge of their seat deeply fixated on the next captivating detail of this challenging birth. That wasn't enough. The suspense increased as other mothers now who 'previously' said they had a manageable birth, added extra juicy tip bits to their birth stories. Now it seemed a competition was on who could win and be crowned 'the Mother Group's most traumatic birth!'

Years later, when we catch up, our birth experiences still feature as part of the conversation. It seemed the only ones who are still doing the talking are those who had the difficult births. I have noticed over time that the mothers who were traumatised by their birth feel the need to talk through it again and again and again, often with anyone who will listen. Studies have shown that people who have what they class as traumatic birth experience, tell on average thirty-five people about it. Those who have a good birth experience, tell just twelve.

Women find the need to discuss their challenging birth experience in order to get a sense of therapy from it. Most don't see counselors about their birth experiences, as they are incorrectly told that bad birth experiences are normal, and you should be happy that there is a 'healthy mother and baby'.

As a society, we don't tend to help those mothers who feel disempowered by birth. Therefore, the only way a women feels that she can get any type of therapy and release from her pain is to talk and talk about her birth experiences. In addition, as her civic duty, she will do what she can to warn other mothers of the horrors of birth. As a result, our view of birth in our society is getting an unbalanced with negative beliefs about birth. The next time you meet someone so keen to share their bad birth story with you; have a heart and think about what they went through. Then take a deep relaxing breath and mentally thank yourself for choosing a different, positive birth experience for you and your baby.

Our birth motivation affects how we birth

A fifteen year old teenager had disguised her pregnancy from her friends and family. She went to school one day as usual and during class, she excused herself and went to the bathrooms to have her baby, quickly, quietly and without the knowledge of others. Her concern over being detected created a far stronger motivation than any fear she may have had of the birthing. And so her baby was born easily and in very little time, without any discomfort. She then proceeded to go back to class, and remarkably carried on the rest of the school day, before picking up the baby from the bathroom later in the day.

Most of us wouldn't dream of giving birth in public toilet or wish for these extreme birth circumstances. Interestingly though, she seemed to have a strong belief in her ability to birth easy and effectively. During her birth, her mind never accepted, or even considered, that there would be any impediments to this birth or that she would experience the long, typical labor that our society has come to expect.

Do you really want a 'boring birth'?

If we think back to my example from my mothers' group, we ask: What was each of these women's birth motivations? Was there deep down, a need to have the worst possible birth experience? Perhaps to feel validated for going through a life changing experience? A story of trauma that would be played out at dinner parties for the next ten years? Perhaps there's a position of power to hold over our partner's heads for a long time to come?

I remember hearing a father say to his three year old, 'Now be nice to mommy, as she went through a lot when you were being born.' Remember the Seinfeld TV show where George's obnoxious mother screamed about being in labor for forty-eight hours to manipulate George's actions?

Is there a **secondary benefit** in us when we birth? Are we secretly, perhaps somewhere deep down, wishing for a traumatic birth experience, so we can get some more air time or credibility with our friends and family? I know it might seem a strange suggestion for a course on natural birthing.

 Quick Exercise:

*Stop for just a moment, take a deep breath and honestly ask yourself if there is **some benefit** to having an edge of the seat, action packed, sensational birth story, where you all eyes are focused on you, lapping up all the attention?*

You might find that there is just a strong need for attention and sensation in your life - **this is normal**. Think of the most popular TV shows on at the moment. They are mainly 'reality TV' where we enjoy the tears, the tantrums, the turmoil and the twists and turns. These shows are classed as 'boring' if they are focused on happy, pleasant, harmonious relationships and interactions. Take a moment to think about all the shows on TV, from the drama to the documentaries and you will find that all have the ingredients of intrigue to make it more entertaining for us to watch.

As we are naturally drawn to the drama in a situation, you may think that birth is different. Well, what are you watching on TV right now about birth? The shows, 'One born every minute,' the Discovery Health's 'Deliveries' and 'Special Care Babies,' these all follow the same rule to adding drama to our viewing. What do we find more gripping and involving: the easy, birth with a smile or the mother who is extreme distress where any moment the baby will be in danger and major intervention is need to save both the mother and the baby? Well, like most of you, I tended to be magnetized to the more traumatic birth experience, unfortunately.

We are **hard wired to feel empathy and a connection to those who are in distress**. We are almost mesmerized into watching more and more of these types of programs. The problem with watching these scenes is we start to automatically identify ourselves with the person who had the challenging birth and then because we are feeling empathy. Our mind then connects with the program and we start to put our own self in this challenging birth experience. Now you are thinking, feeling and daydreaming about your own very negative birth experience. We know that **this self-hypnotizing**

process can over time change our beliefs and bring about the experiences into our reality. So be careful what you feed your mind! Focus only on what you wish your birth to be.

Monitor what you feed your mind

I had to ban myself from watching 'Terrifying Twin Deliveries' on TV. I justified to myself that this was education and I was purely watching the shows to be informed. In reality, I was watching the shows to feel connected to the drama and intrigue. It took me awhile to piece together the connection that watching these shows had on my belief to have an amazing birth. I started slowly at first to doubt my own ability to birth naturally and my fears started to creep slowly back into my mind. The amazing and beautiful birth that I had dreamed about and claimed as my own, started to dissolve and my daydreams were replaced with fear, intervention and suffering.

The only way to reclaim my rightful birth was to ban all these traumatic birth shows from my mind. I hired DVDs on beautiful natural birth and surfed YouTube for more hypnobirthing births. Every day, I watched at least one short beautiful birth to remind myself on a daily basis of the amazing ability of my body to perfectly birth my babies in the most fulfilling adventure of my life. I can tell you the feeling of knowing you have given birth naturally is such an overwhelming and significant experience. This birthing day is one day that will stay in your memories for the rest of your life.

When I spoke to my mothers' group about my birth and was dismissed for having a 'boring birth,' I can fundamentally tell you that my twins 'birth was the absolute best 'boring birth' in the entire world.

When it comes time for your Hynobirth, the euphoria of that moment will resonate within your soul for your entire life. That experience, can never even come close to your '15 minutes of traumatic birth fame'. Choose which birth experience you truly wish to have and choose wisely. And then do all you can, to make your birthing day one that you claim as your own piece of history.

OVERCOME YOUR FEARS AND HAVE AN AMAZING BIRTH

If you are like most pregnant women, you will find that as you move through these days and months of pregnancy, you will be met with a whole new set of feelings, thoughts, doubts, questions, and decisions that you never had to consider before. All these new emotions and decisions will cause you to look at the many transformational experiences that bringing a baby into your life will present. This is natural and normal.

As you prepare your mind and body for your baby's birth, you will want to be free of any fears, reservations, or limiting thoughts. It's helpful for both you and your partner to be able to identify feelings, experiences or recollections that may be painful or hurtful. After all, these could limit your ability to approach birthing free of harmful emotions.

Take a look at those emotions that may foster a feeling of uneasiness and meet them head on and release any conflict you may be holding onto, perhaps even at a subconscious level. Once you have been able to work through and resolve lingering emotions, limiting thoughts, experiences, or memories that could stand in the way of an easy birthing, you will have a better sense of your own ability to approach the birth of your baby with trust and confidence.

It easy to just brushing aside matters that concern you now. This may be OK for the pregnancy, yet at the birth, that is when fears tend to erupt quickly to the surface at your birthing time. This can lead to the fear-tension-pain syndrome and significantly change the course of your birth. Take advantage of the opportunity to talk with your partner, your birthing companion or a good friend who can help you explore and discuss any thoughts that could be troubling you. They may not be able to help you solve them at this time, however listing and acknowledging these issues are a vital first step to clearing them from your life.

Author's Thoughts

'A few years before I had my twins, I worked with Susan, who was due to give birth for the first time in a few months, and she invited all the attention she could find. Susan expected to be waited upon and needed constant pampering. She even said to me that since she is pregnant, she shouldn't have to get her own cup of tea anymore. It started to drive us all a little crazy. Susan believed the concept of pregnancy is an abnormal condition and she is 'ill'. She barely tolerated her pregnancy and constantly proclaims her annoyance at all the aches, pains and other pregnancy "disorders," even though she seemed really healthy.

When I met Susan's mum, I knew where it had all started. She was continually cautioning her daughter, that she must "give in" to her frailty during this precarious time of her life. As it got closer for Susan to give birth, I couldn't avoid the constant conversations about what she expected her birth to like. She recalled in depth the horrendously long and difficult births her mother and all of the women in her family experienced. This was the centerpiece of her conversation week after week. As I got to know others in her family, I saw that all the women in the family talked in "victim" language. Despite the fact that their birth stories were horrific, they were delighted to tell all of the details, each one surpassing the other, and each rushing in to grab her opportunity to tell how bad her pregnancies and birthing were.

I was really amazed when I heard that Susan was planning to have a natural birth and had some natural birth education classes as well. Yet, she appeared to embrace the whole natural birth philosophy and said she was going to put her family's birth past behind her and now she was believing for a natural and easy birth.

I must admit that this was quite a transformation and I did find it a bit surprising that she would make such a change. I was so pleased for her and excited about the easy birth she was now after.

Susan's new found excitement and natural birth belief fizzled out by the end of the week. She was back to the same old conversations of birth horror stories. I really was hoping for an easy birth for Susan, but I was not surprised that her birthing story was one that could easily match and top those of her family members. The drama surrounding the birth was incredible, and there was a gathering of family and friends invited in to observe the performance. It seemed it was more important for Susan to be able to remain in good standing, and meet the birth expectations of her family and friends than it was to remain outside the group and to birth her baby calmly and peacefully as she had prepared. **Kathryn Clark, Author**

For Susan, her true beliefs about birth had been ingrained from such an early age and just wanting to have a natural and easy birth isn't enough. In order for real change to happen, her beliefs, motivation, thoughts and feelings need to be incongruent.

It's important to assess your own motivation and intent as you approach your birthing. Consider how you will apply these Laws of the Mind so that they work for you. Your motivation is closely tied to your desire and self-image. It is said that a woman births pretty much the same way that she lives life. For that reason, it is important that you take the time to assess how you see yourself and whether this image is productive or counterproductive for you and your birth.

'Normal' birth can be traumatic

Making the leap into motherhood can bring about the additional challenges of a postpartum period. Most people know about the baby blues, and the media has given a good deal of attention to postpartum depression (PPD). However, less attention has been given to the unique problems suffered by mothers who experience symptoms that seem like postpartum depression, but the symptoms are more intense.

Research makes it clear that women can suffer extreme distress as a consequence of their experiences during childbirth. A small proportion of pregnancies and births involve events that most people would agree are potentially traumatic. It seems that other women may have what society class as a seemingly 'normal birth,' but feel traumatised by aspects of the birth, such as loss of control, loss of dignity, or the dismissive, hostile or negative attitudes of people around them.

Post-Traumatic Stress Disorder in birth

Recently it has become recognised that women who experienced a traumatic birth (or even what a women perceives as traumatic) can develop post-traumatic stress disorder (PTSD). We once thought that PTSD was reserved for soldier's coming back from war or survivors of horrific experiences. Now we now know that any traumatic experience of birth, can give the same PSTD symptoms. The American Psychiatric Association defines the symptoms of PTSD[10]as:

1. Persistently re-experiencing the event, by flashbacks, nightmares, intrusive thoughts, and intense distress at reminders of the event.

2. Persistent avoidance of reminders of the event, and emotional numbing and estrangement from others.

3. Persistent symptoms of increased arousal. This means difficulty falling or staying asleep, irritability or outbursts of anger, difficulty concentrating, hyper vigilance or an exaggerated startle response.

For a diagnosis, women must report experiencing all three types of symptoms for longer than one month. Many women (around 30% of all births) experience these symptoms in the days or weeks following birth, and this is a normal way of coming to terms with a stressful or overwhelming event. It is only when symptoms do not get better that PTSD is diagnosed (in up to 5% of post-natal women[11]).

The causes of birth PTSD

Research has been carried out into what makes someone more likely to develop PTSD following childbirth. These risk factors fall into three categories[121314]:

1. **Those that exist before the birth:** Some women will be more vulnerable to a traumatic birth because of pre-existing problems. For example, women with a history of psychiatric problems and previous trauma are more likely to be traumatised by their experience of birth. In particular, a history of sexual trauma or abuse is associated with PTSD after birth.

2. **Aspects of the birth itself:** Women are more likely to get PTSD if they have an emergency caesarean or assisted delivery (forceps or ventouse). Importantly, women who feel *out of control* during birth or who have poor care and support from midwives and doctors are more likely to get PTSD.

---

[10]American Psychiatric Association. (2000). *Diagnostic and statistical manual of mental disorders* (Revised 4th ed.). Washington, DC: Author.

[11] Creedy, D.K., I.M. Shochet and J. Horsfall. 2000. Childbirth and the development of acute trauma symptoms: incidence and contributing factors. *Birth* 27(2): 104–11.

[12]Turton, P., et al. 2001. Incidence, correlates and predictors of post-traumatic stress disorder in the pregnancy after stillbirth. *Br J Psychiatry* 178: 556–60.

[13]Wijma, K., J. Soderquist and B. Wijma. 1997. Posttraumatic stress disorder after childbirth: a cross sectional study. *J Anxiety Disord* 11(6): 587–97.

[14]Hofberg, K., and I. Brockington. 2000. Tokophobia: an unreasoning dread of childbirth. A series of 26 cases. *Br J Psychiatry* 176: 83–85.

3. **Support and care women get after birth:** Following the birth, support from friends, family and health professionals may help women resolve their experiences and recover from a traumatic birth. Conversely, a lack of support may prevent recovery or possibly cause more stress and thereby increase symptoms.

Your feelings matter

In some cases, births are mismanaged and a woman can feel challenged to get past her experience. She may go over and over the events in her head and feel angry that she was denied the experience she could potentially have had. This 'reliving' the event can form part of the symptoms of PTSD. A woman who feels very angry is struggling with a valid emotional response to being discounted or not listened to during the birth, or even being feeling mistreated or assaulted. If a women doesn't neatly fit into the "PTSD box" (fulfilling all the symptom criteria), she would still benefit from additional support, counseling or therapy in conjunction with the Hypnobirthing Hub Home Study Course.

 Mother's Thoughts

"With my first birth, Toby, I had a pretty bad birth, and my family just told me to "get over it... what I was complaining about?" I had a healthy baby and that is all that matters, they say. Well, for me, that wasn't enough. I felt robbed and even abused. It got so bad that I kept on having these flashbacks, and feeling I was right there again experiencing the agony all over again. I couldn't even have sex at first, because I saw the hospital staff's faces whenever I had my legs apart.

I wanted another child and I needed to repair the gaping hole in my relationship with my husband and my baby. I sort the help of a pregnancy and birth psychologist and read Lynn Madsen's book 'Rebounding from Childbirth'. That gave me enough strength and peace to start the healing process for another child. I think you are at the right time in your life to find what you need when you really, REALLY want a great birth this time. I remember the quote, 'when the student is ready the teacher will appear'. Hypnobirthing was the teacher for me, and it made the almighty difference in the birth of Chloe.

I remember crying most of the time, as I read through the Hypnobirthing Home Study Course material and sobbing my heart out when listening to the Release All Fear CD. It was just what I needed, when I needed it. Once I got over the flood of tears, I know I was ready, yes really ready now to have my daughter. It was such a contrast to my first overly medicalised birth. This time, I was in a birth center and gave birth in the bath with my husband and two friends. My birth music was in the background as I birthed in calm at my own pace and it was just my birth! I burst into tears when I was handed Chloe, she looked peaceful as she connected to me in an instant. Our eyes were just locked together for ages. It is an experience I will remember forever. I cried with such joy when I held Chloe for the first time, and then a few minutes later, I sobbed and sobbed as I remembered Toby's birth and felt so sad that his birth wasn't like this, yet I felt ok and Chloe's birth was my final healing. I am now at peace. **Jessica Fernandez, California, USA**

Hypnobirthing reduces birth trauma

We are all aiming for a beautiful, natural, fulfilling and empowering birth. For most of us, just by taking the Hypnobirthing Home Study Course and practicing the techniques, we will be able to have this wonderful and powerful birth experience that will last for the rest of our lives.

At the end of the course, we have learnt so many tools to keep the fear and emotions at bay. We would have mastered deep relaxation and breathing techniques in preparation for the birth. We have a thorough understanding of the mechanics and natural stages of birth, and know in advance how we wish our birth to be and this is communicated clearly with our care provider. Our birth preferences are written confidently and concisely on our birth plan. Even our partner feels ready and competent in being a tower of strength and support for us, and is strong, assertive, yet respectful of the medical team.

If a **change of plans occurs**, we simply stop, take a deep breath and relax, and remind ourselves that we are still in control of our birth. And as such, we know what interventions we will be the best in our circumstances. With our birth partners, we use our 'BRAIN' (Unit 4) to ask suitable questions and make informed decisions. So no matter what happens, we are deciding the course of our birth, every step of the way. This is true empowerment.

We are making the decisions, whatever those choices need to be for our health and the health of our beautiful baby. With hypnobirthing, you will find such an inner strength, a power base so strong, solid, impenetrable and immoveable. This is what a fulfilling and empowering birth is really about.

Face your birth fears and beliefs

Take this important step to overcoming any fears or unhelpful beliefs about birth by acknowledging and facing them head on. Bringing them out into the open, writing them down, and talking about them is a huge step forward. This is especially the case for partners, who may never have had the opportunity to speak up in a safe, supported environment about what worries them. It is so often the women's issues and concerns that gains the focus and we forget all together about the partner's fears. It is vital that partner to be a pillar of strength, courage, and conviction, so the mother feels supported, encouraged, and connected to her partner at they join together as one, to bring their baby into their loving family unit.

By bringing your fears up to the surface now, they will not become the lurking "tiger" in the shadows, ready to pounce once you are in the vulnerable state of giving birth, as you will soon realise that **fears are simply thoughts.** They are not concrete activities that will take place for definite: they are simply thoughts derived from the sum of your previous experiences. As with any thought, we can **accept them, let them go and change them for ones that are more useful and beneficial.**

FEAR RELEASE WORKSHEET (BACKGROUND)

Find a quiet time to sit and focus your attention on what is concerning you about your birth. What fears, limiting thoughts, nagging doubts, questions, concerns and changes needing to be made? Think of the effect on your relationship, body, lifestyle, career, income, and responsibilities, parenting styles, doubts or issues from your past. Fill in the work sheet and be as honest as you can. The more open you are about your fears, the less likely they will suddenly rear their ugly head at the birth.

Often, we are told in life to 'just put it out of our mind' and move forward. Unfortunately, birth doesn't work like that. It has this habit of suddenly appearing in labor. I have seen women scream at their partners during birth: 'We can't possibly live in our house anymore!' much to the puzzled look on her partner's face who didn't realise it was a problem and wondering why she is so upset about it now?

Spend time together to reflect

After you have both filled in the fear release worksheet and your partner (and/or someone supporting you through birth) has done the same; agree a time to spend to go through both lists together. Making a date and go out for dinner is a good time to do this. Select a venue where you can give your full undivided attention to each other. Often, just really talking about your concerns can make such a significant difference to alleviate these concerns.

Once you have filled out your fear release worksheet and had your discussion, you may choose to listen to the Hypnobirthing Home Study Course '**Release All Fear of Birth**' Mp3. Through this therapeutic hypnotherapy session, you and your partner will have the opportunity to release many of your concerns already listed and perhaps others that only your subconscious knew about.

Need extra help?

Sometimes, our fears and concerns are very deep and past trauma in our lives affects the way we want to birth. You owe it to yourself and your baby to get the help of a qualified professional who specialize in pregnancy and birth. Psychologists, counselors and hypnotherapists can provide valuable, specific attention to your concerns.

Women who have had previous traumatic birth experiences, PSTD, sexual, emotional or physical assault, or other experiences have found strength and healing through the hands of these professionals. Most importantly, these women who have taken the power out of their trauma often are the ones who have amazing birth experiences. They have worked so hard to claim their rightful birth prize.

Your thoughts, feelings or experiences are a pebble

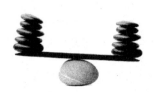 Think of any thought, feeling or experience about birth like a pebble. Anything you heard from childhood until now would be a pebble, anything you saw about birth would be a pebble and anything you experienced or felt about birth would be a pebble. So there would be a lot of pebbles around. Some would be large and these would have a significant impact upon your beliefs and values about birth, whether they are positive or negative. Perhaps some of the larger pebbles may be your own previous birth or that of someone close to you. You will notice there would be many pebbles that are quite small and may seem insignificant. These represent experiences that had some impact, perhaps a movie, a book you read, or a stranger's birth story.

There will be many small pebbles around. While they may seem irrelevant, over time, they will add up and make that difference in your birth beliefs and values. **Your goal is to have more positive pebbles about birth than negatives ones** and with the balance heavily weighted to a positive birth experience. This will make all the difference in having the amazing fulfilling birth within your reach.

Are your scales too heavily weighed down by negative birth beliefs and fears? Not a problem - that is why we are here! The Hypnobirthing Home Study Course will provide all the tools and techniques needed to remove the negative birth pebbles and add to your positive birth pebbles, making your balance heavily on the positive and installing more helpful beliefs about birth.

FEAR RELEASE WORKSHEET

What Was Your Own Birth Like?

What stories have you heard, are they positive or encouraging, or negative and frightening?

What impact do these stories have on your thoughts about your baby's birth?

Do you feel you will duplicate your mother's labor?

To work on: *If what you've been told is less than encouraging, remember you are not your mother, and this is not her pregnancy. You are an entirely different person at a different time and under different circumstances.*

Other Birth Stories

What joyful birthing stories have you been surrounded by?

What negative stories have been passed on to you?

Have family members ingrained you with 'family patterns' of long labors, pain and medical intervention?

What types of birth stories have you been exposed to through the media, internet, stories you've read, and movies you've seen? How have they shaped your thinking on birth?

Have you attended another birth? How has this affected your view on your upcoming birth?

To work on: *It is easy to assume the experiences of the people who are retelling these stories. Yet, there is no reason to believe that you will birth as they did, everyone births differently or there would be no need for women to tell their 'birth stories'. Work at checking what types of thoughts are unhelpful, so that you don't bring someone else's past baggage into your birthing.*

Previous Birthing(s)

Has your own experience with birth been easy and satisfying?

Are you carrying recollections of an arduous ordeal?

Do you need to find healing from this experience?

What do you wish to do differently this time around?

To work on: *If you had a less than satisfying birth, take hope in the fact that you are better prepared for an easier birth this time, and you now can approach birthing with more knowledge and planning than you did before. By using the Hypnobirthing Home Study Course techniques, you will find that the 'sting' from those memories will be gone and you will have a clean slate to have an easy and fulfilling birth this time around.*

Parenting

Did you learn positive attitudes toward parenting that you feel comfortable with? If not, do you feel less than adequate about your ability to be a good parent?

Do you feel overwhelmed with being a parent and the responsibility?

Is your partner's parenting style in agreement with your own?

How would you like to parent this baby? Do you have the skills/resources/support, etc., to do so?

To work on: *Quite often, people who did not grow up with good role models can learn a great deal about what not to do and how they wish for their own children. Turn these desires into a positive factor and use this time to provide healing from the past, so you can be the best parent you can be.*

Support

Do you feel secure with the support that your partner and/or family will provide?

Is there someone who will share the responsibilities of caring for the baby?

How could you get the support you need?

To work on: *Sometimes, just letting people know you want and need support will resolve the matter. Also see what strengths you must build within yourself to effectively provide your own best support.*

Marriage/Relationship

Is your relationship secure, loving and mutually nurturing?

Are you confident that your relationship is strong and that it will weather the additional strain of raising a child?

Are there some agreements or arrangements that you need to work out? Have you really talked about what you think your needs will be?

Will you get the support you need from your partner?

To work on: *By talking and really listening to each other can go a long way in resolving those nagging issues and concerns. This will lay the foundations for a secure relationship when it is challenged by the addition of your baby. Working together on Hypnobirthing can bring about a stronger bond than you ever believed could exist.*

Career

Will you be able to continue to pursue your own goals? Will some reorganizing and planning be needed?

Will your plans need to be put on hold? Are you ok with this change?

Are you apprehensive about going back to work or staying home with your baby?

Does your partner support you in your goals about going back to work or staying home with your baby? How does this affect the relationship?

To work on: *Sorting through these questions can help you feel at peace with what you really feel you want to do and the best for you, your baby, partner, and family.*

Housing

Is there room in your home for your new baby? Can accommodations be easily made?

If your housing is not suitable, what could you do about it?

To work on: *Finding peace in your current circumstances, or see how your circumstances can change and the choices you may need to make.*

Medical Care

Do you feel comfortable with your present medical care provider? What do you like best or least?

Do you feel that he or she is supportive of your hypnobirthing plans for your birthing? Are there lingering doubts?

Have you discussed your preferences for a natural birth with this person and made your wishes known?

Do you think your medical care provider is operating from a 'fear basis' or 'confidence basis'?

Is the rate of intervention for this care provider/facility acceptable for you? How do you think this will affect your birth?

To work on: *When you birth, you need to be fully relaxed and feel supported by those around you, if you don't feel you will be given the care, attention and support that you need, then it is time to change providers.*

Finances

Do you see finances being "stretched" as a result of adding another person into your life?

Does this concern you?

To work on: *Change or find acceptance in your circumstances. Remember the Law of Attraction? This can work with finances, as well. Think positive thoughts of financial plenty.*

Baby Bonding

Do you feel connected to this child?

Are you excited and overjoyed at bringing a new baby into your family?

Are you apprehensive and concerned about the effect this baby will have upon your life?

Are other family members bonded to this child?

To work on: *Connecting to your child is an important piece of the hypnobirthing program, yet sometimes there are blockages that may stop us feeling the love and deep sense of attachment to your child. Listening to the Hypnobirthing Home Study Course Mp3 track 'Quick relaxation and baby bonding' (from pregnancy relaxation and health album) makes a significant difference in resolving those issues, so you can deeply attach to your child.*

Personal Experience of Abuse

Are you holding onto unhappy memories of physical or sexual abuse?

Are any influences from traumatic memories or experiences affecting you?

To work on: *Your body and birthing is one of the most profoundly physical experiences you will know in your lifetime. If these are not addressed and released, they may reappear at your birthing. Overwhelming feelings of helplessness, inadequacy, and fear have the ability to make your body shut* *down or resist. It is important that you do release work with a qualified professional before you advance any further into your pregnancy.*

Please take this assessment seriously. Your mind and body work best when both are in harmony so that you can approach your birthing with peace.

QUICK RELEASE OF YOUR EMOTIONS

Often, we may feel overwhelmed with emotions in our daily lives. Perhaps you have noticed this yourself when you find yourself angry, frustrated, and annoyed, or experiencing other unwanted emotions. We easily find ourselves 'overreacting' to situations even on a daily basis. At other times, the same situation may not have even caused us to raise an eyebrow. This disconnect between what we feel at times can be confusing and may feel we are lost at the mercy of our emotions.

This 'Quick Release' of your emotions is designed for when you need a fast way to deal with an emotional issue. The next time you find that someone's comments have 'wound you up' tighter than a cuckoo clock, just take a deep breath and follow the Quick Release Technique. In time, as you allow yourself to become engaged in the process, you will easily find that you can quickly release any emotion you need in just a few minutes.

*For those who want a guided quick release session. There are three **Quick release tracks** on the Hypnobirthing Home Study Course CD/Mp3 of 'Release all fear of birth'.*

This quick release technique is inspired by the revolutionary Sedona Method[15] and is now adapted to bring you the best way to quickly release your emotions that will arise during your pregnancy and birth.

1.   You are not your feelings or beliefs

The more expectations and ideals about the way that things should or shouldn't be, the more you struggle against what is 'the right now.' People are so often caught up in their emotions that they actually feel they *are* the emotion. We say 'I am angry' rather than 'I am *feeling* angry.' The emotion can feel as if it is part of who we are and our identity, so we find ourselves overly caught up in the experience.

2.   Choose to release your emotions and let go

When you choose to release your emotions and just let go, everything gets easier. Your goals start to manifest because you are actually removing yourself as a blockage out of the way. Decide that this emotion isn't actually you, and you can let it just go. Doing so, we realize that by letting go, we find instant freedom from our emotions and find clarity and emotional maturity. So be free of your emotional hold. Ask yourself: Are you in charge of your emotions or your emotions in charge of you?

What do you mean by letting go?

 Quick Exercise: **Pick up a pen or a pencil.**

For the sake of this exercise, the **pen** that you're holding represents your *unwanted emotions* and also your beliefs about yourself. All those unwanted things that are holding you back. And your **hand** represents your awareness. Take the pen and grip it as tight as you can with your hand. Now if we did

---

[15]H. Dwoskin, The Sedona Method: your key to lasting happiness, success, peace and emotional well-being. Sedona Press, 2003

this long enough, it would start to feel really uncomfortable and then actually ok. The series of being uncomfortable then feel ok is what we're doing all the time with our emotions.

Now open your hand and roll the pen around in your hand. Is the pen attached to your hand? No, obviously not. But if you think about your emotional experience, most of the time it feels like it's attached to you. Our emotions, our beliefs, feel like *they are us*. But every emotion you have, every belief you have, all the things you're struggling with are attached to you as this object is attached to your hand.

Now close your hand lightly around the pen and release and *just let it go*. Just like the pen, your emotions fall away. That's what we mean by releasing and letting go. It's really that simple. Allowing what is to be, embracing life and allow feelings to pass through you like clouds through the sky

Blockages to releasing and letting go

Sometimes, we hold so tight to our emotions and feel justified in keeping these emotions close to us. We won't allow ourselves to be free of the emotions. Your name tag is stamped all over them. These emotions could be directly related to birth or something you think is totally unrelated. No matter the source of the issue, if you are feeling emotions of anger, fear, rejection, grief or guilt, they all affect your chemical makeup in your body and your baby.

Remember the 'Mind Body Connection'? If you are feeling an emotion, your baby is as well. It is important to do what you can to free yourself of any unhelpful emotion and give your baby the best possible start.

While we wish to give our baby the best pregnancy experience, I can hear justifications for holding on to your emotions. *"I want to hate my obstetrician, because he ....." "I will always remember what she said to me...." 'It was inexcusable what went on, it will haunt me forever..."* It's as if our justifications will protect us from flooding our body with harming negative emotions. In addition, by holding tight to our emotions, this will somehow 'punish' those who did us wrong. Most of the time, the only ones being 'punished' are ourselves. The emotion is gripping us, holding us so tight, that we're wound up its grasp and unable to break free. Yet all the while we think 'our perpetrator' is the one, not us, being bound and held captive.

The reasons we block ourselves from letting go

1.   Everyone holds onto a lot more than they are letting go.

We believe that we are the only ones in the world and this personal 'me' should be able to control the actions of others and circumstance. It is 'me' against the world. So we constantly resist the way it actually is because it's not the way we planned it.

2.   The mind separates everything into polarities

What we perceive as good, we keep close by and what we perceive as bad, far away from us. When you welcome both polarities and start to accept some grey into your life, the polarities dissolve each other.

3.   We prefer to hold onto our suffering

Ask yourself the question "Would I rather hold on to this suffering or would I rather let go and feel free?" Start the process by welcoming what is, allow it to be there, then follow your heart. If you're struggling with releasing, you can put your hand on your heart to help you get more in touch with what you're experiencing.

4.   When we want to change what is

When we wish things to be different, we recreate the experience in our minds over and over again until we think we can actually change the past. When you let go of wanting to change something, you simply change what you can and allow the rest to be as it is. Always being in a 'wanting' state does not allow us to appreciate life or enjoy it for what it is. As you let go of wanting to change, things get more harmonious and easier.

5.   When we want to figure it out

Many times, the only thing holding a problem in place is our wanting to figure it out and when you insist on a reasonable answer. It keeps you stuck. The only reason we want to understand our problems is because we are planning to have them again. Pause for a moment to think about it. When you let go of wanting to figure it out, you open yourself to clear reason and intuitive knowingness. Insights are helpful, but what's more powerful than trying to have an insight, is to let go first. You don't need to hold on to your suffering until you figure it out. Often, when you take yourself and your emotion out of the situation, the dust will settle and bring a new clarity of thought and understanding.

THE QUICK RELEASE TECHNIQUE

The first step to releasing an emotion is to welcome it in. It might seem a little counterintuitive to welcome in something that you are planning getting rid of. Yet, our emotion have continually been buried within us and by bringing them to the surface and allowing them to gain your attention, is a very effective way of addressing the situation and accepting what is now.

This welcoming is a simple process, which allows us to get in touch with our emotions quickly and effectively.

1.   Welcome the issue: the thoughts, feelings, beliefs or whatever you are experiencing.
2.   Welcome any desire to do something about it, such as fix it or understand it.
3.   Welcome any sense of identity you have with the issue. That it is personal.
4.   Ask yourself, can I release it and just let it go?
5.   **Then simply close your eyes and count 1,2,3,4, then say 'Release' on a long out breath** (and just feel the emotion floating away from you)*.
6.   Repeat this process as many times until the emotion has gone.

Step 5. Simply count 1,2,3,4 and saying "release" does sound too simple to work. Yet, it does work if you continue to use this process. In time, you will easy associate this simple action with emotional freedom. Each success from releasing emotions will anchor your continued ability to find peace and comfort.

If an emotion takes a hold of you, you will simply stop wherever you are, follow the Quick Release process in your mind and cut yourself free of the emotional hold.

EMOTIONAL RELEASE TOOLS

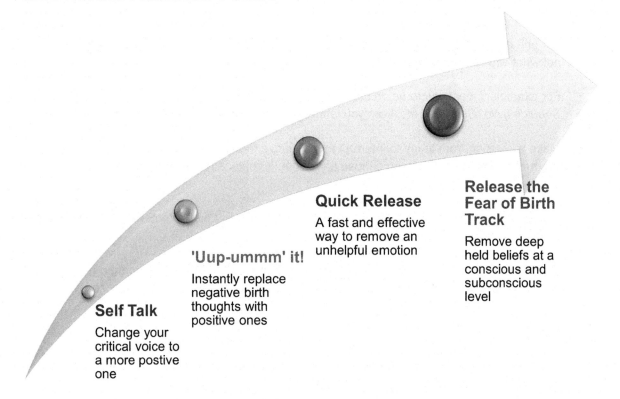

Release the Fear of Birth Track

Remove deep held beliefs at a conscious and subconscious level

Quick Release

A fast and effective way to remove an unhelpful emotion

'Uup-ummm' it!

Instantly replace negative birth thoughts with positive ones

Self Talk

Change your critical voice to a more postive one

UNIT 2: SUMMARY

- **In hypnosis**, your subconscious mind is receptive and is therefore much more likely to succeed in making changes to your beliefs about births. This is far more effective than just relying on determination and willpower.

- **Your Self Talk is a key** to control your emotions. By learning to control your thoughts, keeps you focused on more positive birth images and creates a happier, more balanced emotional experience. 1. Swap 2. Replace and 3. Accept.

- When you think of the **formation of a new belief** as a set of scales, the tipping point is 51%. You will need to be thinking and feeling positive about your birth, more than negatively to install new helpful beliefs.

- **Interrupt** your thoughts, feelings, or daydreams about bad birth outcomes. Find your own way of stopping these thoughts quickly **and replace** them with more positive ones.

- It's essential that you keep your **thoughts and language focused** on what you do want rather than creating wasted negative energy around circumstances that you don't want. Tune into only positive thoughts, feelings and language and feel the difference in your emotions.

- If you are feeling **fear and anxiety** at your birthing time, then adrenaline will be released into your body, causing your surges to stop or slow. Only when you are calm again, will this be a signal for your body to stop the flow of adrenaline and resume labor once more.

- Clearing your fears and emotions are vital to the success of your birth. By being emotionally free, relaxed and calm leads to effective birthing muscles and comfortable birthing.

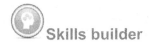

Skills builder

- For one day, see if you can only speak in positive terms. Say what you want to happen and not what you want to avoid.

- For example '*I want you to be on time*' instead of '*don't be late*'. Remove *Not, Don't, Wouldn't, Shouldn't, No, Can't and etc.* from you language for one day.

- Make a decision from today to interrupt any negative thoughts about birth with the **'uup-ummm'** or something else you choose and instantly replace negative birth thoughts with positive ones.

- Monitor any self-talk that is unhelpful for your pregnancy and birth. Remember your baby picks up on the emotions that you feel.

- Gain confidence in the Quick Release technique without the need of the recordings and find emotional freedom easily and instantly.

Partners can help

- You have your own personal baggage around birth. Acknowledge this and understand how this will affect your partner's pregnancy and birth.

- Show your partner you are dedicated to her and the birth by wholeheartedly completing the fear release sheets and recordings.

- She will rely on your calm confidence and a positive mindset during her pregnancy and particularity at the birth. Ensure that you practice all the emotional release tools.

- When she has moments of doubts about the birth, offer to go through an emotional release tool together.

- Encourage her gently to follow the emotional release tools and laws of the mind. Lead by example.

- Being a good birth partner is also about preparing the mind for birth. So start right now!

My mind's prepared for birth: checklist

- ☐ I am more aware of my negative birth thoughts and how this affects my birth outlook.

- ☐ When I have a fear or unhelpful birth thought, I easily find the right emotional release tool to use.

- ☐ I have protected my mind by only hearing positive birth stories, videos, and TV or movies where possible. I am finding it easier to tune out negative birth stories. I know my birth will be my own.

- ☐ Over time, I am finding I have less need to monitor my negative thoughts, they are becoming more positive.

- ☐ I am confident in my birth can be one filled with positivity, joy and peace.

Unit 2: Hypnobirthing Home Study Course Recordings

 Release the Fear of Birth

T1 Introduction
T2 Release all Fear of Birth
T3 Quick Release – Fear
T4 Quick Release – Problems
T5 Quick Release – Relationship

*Listen **once** to all of these recordings and you may need to return to this recording to listen again if required.*

 Audio Guide – Unit 2 (Track 2)

This guide comprises of additional material to support Unit 2 of Hypnobirthing Home Study Course. You can listen once, or as many times as you need. The audio guide is the only recording that you can listen to while you are driving in the car. ***Podcast:*** *For this free audio track on this unit, go to* http://hypnobirthinghub.podbean.com/ *(Episode 4).*

 Videos: **Calm Animal Births**

Have a look on YouTube (or other video sites) for animal births in the wild. By watching these calm, easy and pain-free births; it seems to cement our thinking to how our births are meant to be. When we begin to change our thinking, we too can birth the way nature intended.

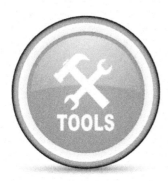

UNIT 3: I HAVE THE TOOLS FOR BIRTH

There's one big secret you must know at this point: The key to your hypnobirthing success is relaxation. The more relaxed you are for each stage of birth, the easier and faster your body will complete the birthing task. In this unit, we learn deep relaxation triggers, visualization and techniques which will enable you to remain relaxed and comfortable at your birth. We focus on the three hypnobirthing breathing techniques, essential when the time comes to birth. There is also a section just for birth partners to keep them prepared, relaxed and confident in knowing the best ways to support you.

HYPNOBIRTHING BREATHING FOR AN EASIER BIRTH

In hypnobirthing, there are three types of breathing uses for the different stages of labor. By using each breathing technique at the right stage, there will be a positive difference in giving you an easy, comfortable and rewarding birth.

1. **Relaxation Breathing**. This breathing is simply to induce a sense of calm and relaxation. It is ideal to implement in pregnancy, the very early/pre labor stages, and in between surges. This technique will instantly bring you to a relaxed state indeed.
2. **Surge Breathing**. This technique in breathing is ideal when you are in established birthing for each surge (contraction). By breathing in this unique way, it reduces any strong sensations to a very manageable level. The technique also makes each surge more effect to thin and open your cervix. This way, you can often reduce your birthing time.
3. **Birth Breathing**. This specific breathing technique is very helpful when you are actually birthing your baby. By working effectively with your body, your baby's entrance into the world is a safe, natural, easy and calm. With birth breathing, you are sure to attain a comfortable and an enjoyable birthing experience.

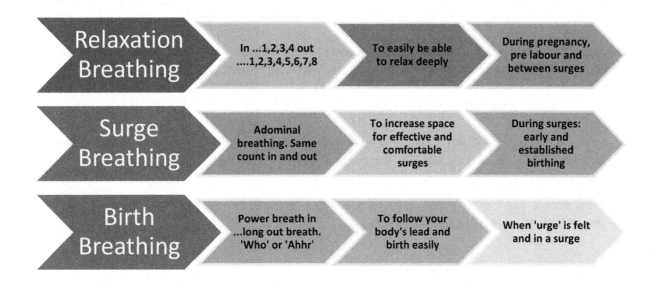

No matter what's going on ....just relax!

It could be just the first twinges of a 'something might be happening.' Or it could already be the crowing of your baby's head. No matter what is going on in the birth process, it is absolutely vital for you to be relaxed at all times.

Here's how relaxation makes such a difference to your birth ....

- Your uterus muscles are free of tension. Being so, it can work much more effectively, therefore **you birth in less time**. There is a very delicate balance between feeling stressed and muscle tension in birth. Even a little tension can cause the uterus muscles to have less oxygen, so the surges are less effective. When this happens, it can slow down or even stop labor. It can also make the birth much longer and more challenging.
- As you will be relaxed in your birthing time, **your baby will also be relaxed**. Your blood pressure and pulse will be low. Your baby's blood pressure and pulse also stay at just the right level. Therefore, your baby is much less likely to become distressed. Unfortunately baby distress is the most common reason for medical intervention. However by being relaxed in your birthing time, you are one step closer to your amazing birth.
- Breathing deeply and rhythmically creates a sense of **calmness and confidence**. You feel so much more present and connected to the birth. As you are so focused, you can easily use all the valuable hypnobirthing tools and techniques. The result is a much easier and fulfilling birthing that you so deserve.

RELAXATION BREATHING

The Relaxation Breathing technique is used for the *early stages* of birthing. It is applied to induce relaxation and calm, perhaps when the surges are just starting. It is also useful *between contractions*, particularly if you need extra relaxation. This technique could also be used whenever you need to create a sense of relaxation *during your pregnancy*. While we know and understand how important it is to be relaxed in your birthing time, it must be learned. Yes, relaxation is a skill to be learned!

Understand that relaxation is impossible in a stressful situation. Ever seen a midwife or doctor almost yelling at a woman in her birthing time *'to just relax'*? Usually the response is *'I can't!'* or *'I just don't know how!'* You can't relax just because you are told to relax or want to relax. It's just impossible, given the stressful condition. Well, for most people that is true. But for **hypnobirthing women, being**

able to relax when or where, no matter what the circumstance or environment, is entirely possible.

In hypnobirthing, we learn to relax easily whenever needed. The relaxation breathing, along with the relaxation and release cues you will later learn, you will be able to feel so deeply relaxed in an instant.

Quick Exercise: *Close your eyes a take a long breath-in through your nose and then a long breath out through your nose. Repeat this three times. Is the in-breath or out-breath more relaxing?*

Most people say the out-breath is more relaxing. Therefore, in relaxation breathing, we make our out-breath twice as long as our in-breath.

Relaxation breathing and early twinges

Before I had my babies, I thought I would know for sure when it was my birthing time and when it was just practice labor. Funny, but on TV, they always seemed to know. In reality it is often a blur between the first twinges and the more established labor. If you are in the *'I'm not totally sure stage,'* then Relaxation Breathing works like a charm. By being so relaxed from the beginning lays the foundation for a relaxed birth. The key here then is to **begin the way you would like to go on.**

Relaxation breathing and in between surges

You now know it is *'the real deal.'* You are having regular surges and performing your surge breathing with each contraction. Now you have some time out before the next surge begins. This *'in between time'* is a time that fears or anxiety can creep in little by little. Perhaps an off handed comment by a caregiver or your partner may have given you a certain look. No matter how well the intentions of people around you during your birthing time, they may just happen to say or do the wrong thing.

Because we birth like mammals, we have such a primal response at our birthing time. In fact, our instincts are overly heightened and we feel **very sensitive at this time**. Yes, you can't control everyone and everything around you during your birth. But you can **easily control your own emotions** and create a sense of calm whenever you need it. If you ever feel you could do with some extra relaxation in the *'in between time,'* just take a few relaxation breaths. When you do that, you'd feel renewed and confident once more.

Relaxation breathing for a calm pregnancy

It is so easy to allow your mind to run away on its own during pregnancy. Even if there is something concerning, you know that any emotion will transfer to your baby. With relaxation breathing, you are able to remain calm, focused and positive. More importantly, the technique gives you the ability to cope with a situation or circumstance. Using the relaxation breathing to stay calm is one of the most important things you can do for your baby right now.

Relaxation Breathing Technique

1. Allow your eyelids to gently close.

2. Consciously drop and relax your jaw, neck and whole body.

3. Slowly inhale through your nose (or mouth) to the count of 4
    Breathe in 1,2,3,4

3. Slowly exhale through your nose (or mouth) to the count of 8
Breathe out 1,2,3,4,5,6,7,8

4. On the out breath, allowing your breath to drift down into the chest, stomach and down through the entire body. Feel your shoulders sink into the frame of your body.

5. Repeat four times or as needed to feel wonderfully relaxed.

Quick Exercise: *Tense only your nose. It is a challenge to tense just your nose. Now in comparison, tense your mouth.*

We find it easier to tense our mouth and this tension then continues to our jaw and down to our neck and shoulders. Our aim in hypnobirthing is to be relaxed as possible. If you are able, breathe in and out through your nose when practicing this breathing exercise. If you have difficulty breathing with your nose, it is okay to breathe through your mouth. Be consciously aware to relax your mouth at all times.

Practice until it is automatic

- It is so important to start relaxation breathing now and continue throughout your pregnancy. Do get used to this unique breathing technique until it becomes second nature to you. This is one exercise we continue, and hopefully, you will never stop as it is a wonderful tool for life.
- You will know when it is second nature, when a difficult moment arises and you automatically just take a relaxation breath and calm yourself.

SURGE BREATHING (CONTRACTIONS)

Relaxation during a surge

A vital step towards reducing strong sensations during childbirth is to learn how to **breathe deeply into your abdomen. With such breathing you must learn how to relax your body to a point that your uterus is free of any unhelpful tension.**

The sensations of birthing are the result of a normal, healthy body function. By allowing your body to do its job, and by accepting and recognizing the sensations of each surge as productive and positive, you also reduce the sensations to a **very manageable level**. In fact, so many hypnobirthing women have reported that they felt comfortable sensations in their birthing time, and there was no pain at all.

When it comes to having a surge, you don't need to learn any complicated breathing patterns. The more you can follow what your body is asking of you, the more likely you are to breathe effectively. Surge breathing **feels right and natural** when you are in a pressure sensation of a surge. You can actually feel the benefits of breathing in this way because it's so intuitive. Plus it makes the surges feel so much less intense and much more manageable.

Surge breathing is abdominal breathing

Ever wondered how free divers can hold their breath underwater for up to seven minutes? So why are most of us gasping for air after thirty seconds? The secret to free diving is to increase your lung capacity and deeply fill your lungs with oxygen. So, how does the free diving sport relate to pregnancy when it's not on the recommended pregnancy exercise lists?

Throughout each surge, the more you breathe steadily, evenly and deeply down to your diaphragm, the better it will be for you and your baby.

Quick Exercise: *Place one hand on your chest and another on your stomach and relax as much as you can. Now don't attempt to make any effort. Just note it down: Do you naturally breathe into your belly or into your chest?*

Some people will find they are breathing into their stomach only and most will find they are naturally breathing into their chest. Some will realize their breathing patterns are a mixture of both.

Note that in 'relaxation breathing,' we don't focus on where you breathe, as it is more an effortless breathing technique. However with surge breathing, it is important to **breathe into your stomach**. This is so you can lessen your pressure sensations during a surge and **connect to a deeper relaxation**.

Deep breathing into your chest is hard work

If you deeply breathe with your rib cage, as you inhale, your rib cage is contracting and you have to move the heavy ribs upwards. And this will take more energy and bring you and your baby less oxygen. Alternatively, during a surge, deeply breathe with your belly. The breath gets slower and deeper, so **you use less energy and get more oxygen**. The more oxygen you breathe in a surge, the better for you, your muscles and your baby.

Abdominal breathing deepens your relaxation

Not only do you have more oxygen and less energy in abdominal breathing, it also creates feelings of relaxation and well-being. Every time you inhale into your belly, the diaphragm is moving down. That is why your belly is bulging out and this movement massages all the internal organs.

When you exhale, the diaphragm is moving up and massages the solar plexus, which is an important nerve center and **enhances our feelings of well-being**. Every time we exhale, we are creating deep relaxation in our body. This type of relaxation is very important when we are at our birthing time. And so we can make every surge as effective as possible to thin, soften and open our cervix faster.

Breathing reduces the pressure sensations of a surge

When you breathe deeply into your abdomen during a surge, you expand your abdomen and lungs. Deep breathing also gives the *vertical muscles* of the uterus more room to reach down and *pull up* the circular muscles. **This extra room for your uterus muscles reduces the intensity of the surge and makes it easier to manage.**

There is a direct link between the more you can breathe up into your abdomen, the easier the pressure sensations of surge will be for you. Therefore, it is important to practice and continually challenge yourself to breathe as deeply and for as long as you can into your abdomen. Over time, this will train your lungs to expand and gain more oxygen so you can easily breathe deeply and longer into your abdomen. Remember the free divers? Yes, that's how it works for them!

All babies breathe with their bellies. Take a quick peek, next time you see a little baby sleeping. This abdominal breathing is preserved in our cell memories; we just need to restore it.

During a contraction, you naturally become very focused on your breathing: you listen to it and observe it, so that you can deliberately ensure it is calm, rhythmic and deep. This kind of belly breathing is synonymous with relaxation. As you are aware, relaxation is the key to a comfortable birth experience. By listening to your breathing and keeping it steady, rhythmical, and deep, you keep tension away - **with no tension, the uterus can do its job far more effectively**.

Ever laughed so much you wet your pants?

Oh, that feeling when we laugh so much. Remember those moments? No doubt, you relaxed, happy and probably had a huge grin with your mouth open wide. These are the perfect conditions to open sphincters in our body. Sphincters???

Ina May Gaskin, the mother of modern midwifery, coined the phrase *'Smile for your sphincter?'* Your sphincters include your excretory (anus and urethra), cervical, and vaginal circular muscles that are responsible for opening, closing and releasing elements from your body. Your sphincters will *open easily* when you are relaxed, at peace and even happy. Ever wondered why constipation is often associated with stress? Yes, that's it!

Sphincters open when we are relaxed, happy and calm and also *can close* when we feel we are being watched, judged, frightened or upset. The *rush of adrenaline* in our bloodstream causes the sphincters to stay closed. That is why we prefer to use the bathroom in privacy and be relaxed.

Another interesting fact about sphincters is they **open best when we open our mouths**. This is why many people wet their pants when they laugh so much! The anus is also a sphincter. The next time open to your mouth, smile and relax when you are doing a bowel movement and notice the difference.

Quick Exercise: *Relax your face and jaw, and open your mouth and throat, and notice what happens.*

When you relax your jaw, open your mouth and your throat. Your bottom automatically relaxes and sinks into your chair. You may even feel you need to go to the bathroom.

'Smile for your sphincter' ... and birth better

Your cervix and your vagina are both sphincters. They need the right conditions to open and allow your baby to pass through easily.

- Open your mouth when you are in surge. Doing so will open your cervix.
- Open your throat when you are birthing your baby. It will open the vagina.
- Create an atmosphere of privacy.
- Relaxation is vital.
- Ensure you are confident in birthing your baby and have overcome any fears.

Benefits of surge breathing

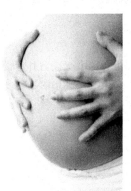

Apart from the emotionally and mentally calming effects of abdominal breathing, you will benefit your birth in many ways. Here are the advantages.

- Creates room for the uterine muscles to be more effective.
- Reduces the intensity of the surge and makes it easier to manage.
- Your blood pressure remains at a healthy level.
- Opening your mouth slightly, helps to open and relax the cervix.
- Increases oxygen to your uterine muscles and to your baby.
- You increase the level of oxytocin (hormone responsible for

regulating contractions).

- Increases the level of prostaglandin (the hormone which softens the cervix).
- Increases the level of relaxin (hormone for stretching the perineum).
- This increases the level of endorphins (the hormone that dulls the sensations in the part of the brain which registers pain).
- Significantly reduces the likelihood of the 'Fear-Tension-Pain' syndrome, leading to 'failure to progress' and the interventions that follows.

> By breathing this way in a surge, it will make the contraction more effective by thinning and opening the cervix faster. The breathing will allow you to lessen the feeling of strong sensations and enable you to manage them more effectively.

Surge breathing - practice technique

1. Relax in a seated position. Your body is relaxed, loose and limp, and your mouth is open.

2. Place your middle fingers just touching on your belly button. Make sure that just the middle fingers will touch.

3. Take a long, slow and deep *breath in* through your nose into your abdomen, breathing up as far you can.

4. As you *breathe in* your fingers will come apart. Note that the deeper the breath, the farther away your fingers will become.

5. Then slowly *breathe out* through your mouth as your fingers return to the just touching again.

6. Slowly *breathe in* for as long as you can to reach a comfortable number. Perhaps 10? Remember; do not hold your breath! You and your baby need oxygen.

7. Slowly *breathe out* to the same count.

8. Slowly *breathe in* 1,2,3,4,5,6,7,8,9,10 (*or what feels right for you*).

9. Slowly *breathe out* 1,2,3,4,5,6,7,8,9,10 (*or what feels right for you*).

10. Continue to breathe in this way for five in and out breaths.

This may feel quite hard work at first. But the more times you practice, the easier it will become. By practicing, you can comfortably increase the count, and this will increase your lung capacity.

Checklist for practicing surge breathing

☐ Are you are breathing from abdomen and not your chest? Look in the mirror and notice that only your stomach is inflating like a balloon and deflating again. If your shoulders and upper chest are rising, you will need to focus breathing only from your abdomen.

☐ While you are at the mirror, note this down: Are your shoulders, neck, and jaw relaxed and free of tension?

☐   Are you breathing in through your nose and out through your mouth? If you wish to breathe only with your nose or your mouth, that is perfectly OK. The main point is to keep your mouth slightly open and relaxed during surge breathing.

☐   Is it your deep and full breath that is doing **most of the work** in pushing your stomach to rise? There will be some tightening in the abdomen. This is normal and beneficial as you breathe in. Just don't actively use your muscles to push it out. Think of your tummy rising and falling like filling a balloon (*breathe in*) and deflating a balloon (*breathe out*).

☐   Are you focusing your attention on your baby as you breathe? Perhaps you may like to imagine your baby happy and relaxed as you breathe in and as you breathe out. You can also focus on your cervix thinning, softening, and dilating easily.

☐   As you practice more, are you easily increasing the count? Is your lung capacity expanding and is your stomach rising higher? You will also notice that your fingers are moving apart more as you breathe in, giving you feedback on your progress.

☐   If you feel Braxton Hicks (practice contractions), are you using the time to practice your surge breathing? You will find the sensation of pressure reducing. This will give you confidence that you are doing it right on the day of your birth.

Surge breathing and your birthing day

On the day you birth your baby, you may want to do a few things differently than what you practiced. Or you may want to keep it exactly the same, which is perfectly fine. Perhaps as you are now so efficient at your surge breathing, it has become automatic and you don't need to count or put your fingers on your stomach to monitor your process.

You may like to go to *'your special place'* when you are in a surge. You will learn the deep relaxation trigger to instantly transport you to that special place. By then you learn to quickly find a deep connection to your birth, your partner, and bring your baby into the birthing process with you. If you choose, you will learn this technique in the Hypnobirthing Home Study Course recording *'Relaxation Triggers and Special Place'* within the album 'Release all Fear of Birth'

However, to fully utilize the technique of accessing 'your special place' while you are in a surge, you need to know the surge breathing automatically.

BIRTH BREATHING

Now you are almost there. Your surges have done an amazing job to fully open the circular muscles and the cervix is fully open (*usually ten centimetres*). Now your **relaxin hormone** flows freely and helps the muscles in the birth canal to open. These muscles can spread out and expand to be large enough for a baby to pass through.

Once this happens, the body steps up a gear and the *longitudinal muscles* in your uterus begin to push the baby down into the birth path for you. The baby is now past the cervix and two to three centimetres into the birth path. This is thought to trigger, *'the urge,'* or *"foetal ejection reflex."* This feeling is a natural, instinctive reflex, similar to an overwhelming bowel movement. It's almost impossible to ignore, and to many women it can feel almost pleasurable after the tightening and releasing sensations.

When Hollywood gets it right

This is the birthing part that dramatized TV and Hollywood movies usually get right. In shows or films, the women would proclaim '*This baby is coming NOW! We are staying right here!'* While in reality, we tend to have a lot more warning through our surges that our baby is coming. What the TV is depicting is *'the urge.'* It is an overwhelming desire to birth your baby. It feels almost physically impossible to stop your body delivering your baby for you. It feels so involuntary and you need to just go with your body and let it do its job.

This desire will be the strongest bodily desire that you have ever felt in your life. Think of your most desperate and strongest feeling to do a bowel movement and you will be a little closer to how the urge will make your feel. 'The urge' (*'foetal ejection reflex'*), also called the *'Ferguson reflex'* or *'spontaneous urge to bear down.'* This urge is felt in birthing mothers who have **natural and non-medicated births**.

Recall again some of the births on TV with 'the urge' - they are usually very quick and uncomplicated from this point on. That is because once you have got to this stage, the birth is almost over. Her body has been working effectively and naturally to bring about this end stage. If you listen to and work with your body, it's less likely that there will be complications from now on. You are on the last stage and often birth can be a quick as a few minutes to thirty minutes.

Be patient for 'the urge'

It is really important to know that there can often be a lull or gap in, or slowing down of the contractions between being fully dilated and experiencing the 'the urge.' During this time, your baby is getting into the right position and **your body is taking a well-earned rest** before the final part of the birth. By trusting your body and allowing 'the urge' to come naturally, your body will do the rest.

It's important not to be hurried into pushing. There is no benefit at all in forced pushes as it could bring potential harm to your body. All you need to do is follow your body's lead and work with your body, gradually and gently assisting your baby into the world.

When Hollywood gets it wrong

Unfortunately, the picture we mostly see on TV is a women lying flat on her back, with the midwife or doctor coming in, checking if she is fully dilated, and looking at the monitor for contractions, then stating '*it is time to push now.'* So we begin to think this 'staff directed pushing' is the normal way to have our baby and we don't need to trust our body to birth our baby for us and wait for 'the urge.' I am surprised to hear that so many mothers to be have never even heard of 'this urge.' It is sad to hear that is this vital part of natural birthing information is being lost.

Interventions will stop 'the urge'

To be fair to our medical staff, most women these days do need to be told when to push. Pardon? I hear you say. That is because many women who birth in hospitals around the world would have had some medical intervention.

You will not get 'the urge' if you have:

- An epidural
- Narcotics (*pethidine, morphine, etc.*)
- Syntocinon or Pitocin (*for inductions and to 'speed up' labor*)
- Staff directed pushing at dilation

These interventions will interfere with your delicate hormone balance in birth and as such, a mother **will not feel the urge** to bear down. This is why her body won't actively birth her baby. It will need additional assistance by pushing her baby out. Even with intervention, the surges are helping the baby to be born; it will just need extra pushing assistance from you. See the 'Perfect Pushing Technique.'

 Doctor's Thoughts

"A woman just the other day, had an epidural and then she just remembered the concept of hypnobirthing of 'breathing her baby out.' She confidently stated that although she had her epidural, she wanted to do it 'naturally' from now on. She won't be allowing any more vaginal examinations and she will wait for 'her natural urge to bear down.' She said her body can birth her baby and she is happy to wait for that to happen.

I am a big supporter of Hypnobirthing, but I must admit, I had a tough time explaining to her, that once the intervention occurs, her birthing hormones are shot to pieces and she will just not get that urge...ever! She has to push when we tell her and it is an endurance sport to push a baby out without the benefit of that urge. She had bloodshot eyes by the end of it and was a mess.

There is a difference between your body automatically pushing your baby out for you and you doing all the work yourself. I tell my patients that staff directed pushing is like running 10 miles up hill compared to taking the bus! Be careful if you want intervention, because you are getting more than you bargained for." **Pierre Vandekamp Obstetrician, Netherlands**

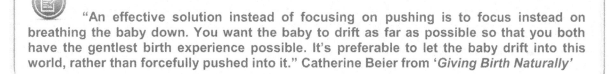 **"An effective solution instead of focusing on pushing is to focus instead on breathing the baby down. You want the baby to drift as far as possible so that you both have the gentlest birth experience possible. It's preferable to let the baby drift into this world, rather than forcefully pushed into it." Catherine Beier from *'Giving Birth Naturally'***

Birth breathing or pushing?

In Hypnobirthing we talk about 'breathing your baby out,' not forcefully pushing your baby out. For some mothers, their body calls out for some assistance in gently pushing (*assisting*) their baby out. For other mothers, they just respond to their body by only breathing the baby down without pushing at all. If you are relaxed and in tune with your body, then follow your body's lead - it will tell you what to do.

I am told to push! NOT breathe...help!!!

With so many women these days having medical intervention and needing coaching in pushing, 'the urge' won't be coming. Therefore, it is becoming common place for medical staff to automatically check to see if she is fully dilated and then instruct her to push her baby out. This can happen even when a women is having a natural birth. And if she agreed to 'staff directed pushing,' she could be end up turning her wonderful natural birth into a medical situation. So, if you are told to start pushing, please say *'I am going to wait for my natural birthing urge and trust my body to birth my baby for me.'*

In addition, make it clear in your birth preferences sheets that you will be following hypnobirthing and will be using mother directed birthing.

A general reminder: When we talk about 'pushing' in a negative way, we mean **'forced pushing' or 'staff directed pushing.'** It is good to be clear about the difference between the two.

Birth breathing	Forced pushing
Waiting for your 'urge'	Don't wait for the 'urge' (or had intervention)
Respond to your body and instinctively *'do what it says'* – follow its lead	Wait for staff to tell you what to do and how to do it.
Relax your pelvic floor muscles when birthing	Tighten and push with all muscles (pelvic floor tight)
Assist your body only as much as it needs (like doing a bowel movement)	Actively push with all your might and effort
Breathing in all the oxygen needed for you and your baby	Told to hold breath and push down hard
Just breathe and follow your body	Count the length of a push
Opens and relaxes your mouth and throat, so your vagina is open and relaxed	Clenches her mouth and jaw, in an effort to push as hard as she can
Breathing relaxes the mother and baby and both are calm during the process	Mother appears stressed and finds it challenging to cope with the experience
Shorter stage: average 10 -20 minutes	Pushing stage longer: average 20 - 40 minutes
Less likely to tear – with birthing upright and perineal massage preparation	Tearing and episiotomy more likely
Assisted delivery unusual, as shorter stage. Mother is calm = baby is calm	Vacuum (ventouse) or forceps more likely, as baby in distress as mother can't effectively push
Feels focused and powerful – birthing is easier on her body and her baby	Feel absolutely exhausted – shaking and vomiting, broken vessels common
Overwhelming joy and happiness in achievement of birthing on her own	Exhaustion and shaking can stop early baby bonding
Holding the baby close and feel the connection to her child	Significantly reduces the enjoyment of birthing
Baby is calm and often not crying at birth	Baby is often seems distressed and inconsolable

Mother's Thoughts

'I had a perfect little baby boy on Tues 10th May, 50cm, 3.365kg, after a very quick labor. Went to see midwife in the morning, and discussed my water birth plan and birth plan again. I had some signs labor was building with some more practice surges and the baby dropping with increased pressure.

Anyway, after the check I went from 1cm to 3cm and started some irregular practice surges varying from 20-10mins apart. At 1pm my waters broke, and I started having surges 2 minutes apart. I grabbed the iPod and started playing the hypnobirthing tracks, and told Dunc to drive me to the hospital since his dad was already at our place to look after Ollie. We got in the car, and I would tap on the dashboard to let Dunc know I was having another surge. Anyway, by the time we got to hospital I could feel the pressure of the baby and knew it was close.

I breathed through a surge in the lift, a surge at the delivery suite doors, and a surge at the nurses' station. Before going to the room our midwife had prepared with the bath and I stepped straight in. I almost immediately felt the urge to breathe the baby down. I didn't have the iPod in, but Dunc was behind me supporting me in the bath. Dunc and the midwife encouraged the birth breathing and letting my body bring him down. I breathed through maybe 3-4 surges, eating ice chips in between surges and Fin's head was born about 10 minutes after getting in the bath. This time I really breathed his head out, I didn't push. After his body was born, I caught him and brought him to my chest. We waited for the cord to stop before cutting it later and the placenta came away with little effort. Fin did a little grizzle but was so alert and interested in what was going on and so happy to have cuddles with mum and dad in the bath. Just magical!

I felt so in control and relaxed despite the quick time frame, and was so happy with the whole experience. **Jen and Dunc, Sydney Australia**

The similarities between bowels and babies

As birthing your baby has so many similarities with doing a bowel movement, we can make some crude analogies. I am sure a lesson in going to the bathroom is a strange one in a birth course. Yet it's important to understand just how naturally similar birthing your baby is to going to the toilet.

1. Prepare and relax

You need to actively prepare and relax into a bowel movement and the same is true in birth. Even if you feel you need to go to the toilet, you can choose to wait until a more suitable time. When you are at the toilet and you prepare your body in an **upright position**, making use of **gravity** and then **relax** into the process. Interestingly, how many people do a bowel movement lying down?

Anyway, the same is true for birth. You can choose to ignore 'the urge' and close your body (although it is a challenge to do). It is not that uncommon for women to 'refuse' to give birth until her obstetrician has arrived. The birthing mother simply chooses not to prepare and relax into the process and actively resists her 'urge.'

Once you are mentally and physically prepared for birth, you will need to position yourself in the **best gravity aided birthing position and then importantly *relax* into the birthing process**.

2. Open and encourage

When you are in a bowel movement and are prepared and relaxed, you will need to then *open your bowels and encourage* the movement. Interestingly enough, we never have to teach our babies and children how to have bowel movements; they simply know how to do it. It is a reflex that is ingrained upon us from before birth.

Birth is no different. We have this innate ability to birth our baby without the need for knowledge. All mammals have this **instinctive knowledge**. It is imprinted upon our mind and body. When the time comes, we instinctively know what to do; we just need to quiet ourselves down enough to 'hear' what to do.

How many times have we heard of people birthing their baby all on their own or people who gave birth on the toilet when they didn't know they were pregnant? In addition, women in comas in hospital have easily birthed their baby without anyone noticing!

When you are prepared and relaxed to give birth, you will be **opening together the same muscles we would do a bowel movement and our pelvic floor muscles relax**. Your 'urge' will be strong at this time, and your body will be almost demanding that you open and *gently* encourage these muscles.

3. Gently relax and release your muscles

When you are doing a bowel movement, we all know it can require just the gentlest of assistance of our muscles to release. We also know that if our diet is poor or we are unhealthy, we can create a more 'constipated' feeling. This means we would need more forceful engaging of our muscles to have successful 'release'.

With the aim to birthing your baby like an **easy bowel movement,** you will only need to gently assist your muscles to bring your baby into the world. Your baby will come out very easily and quickly, and your body will do the rest. Conversely, if a woman is unprepared for birth physically, and gives birth in a more reclined position, then she will need to apply much more pressure and effort to assist her body to birth her baby.

Relax your pelvic floor in birthing

We know that it is important to develop good pelvic floor muscles while pregnant. This is so that after the birth, your pelvic floor muscles return to shape much faster. There will be no embarrassing leaking problems when you sneeze, laugh or jump. Equally, it is important to develop a strong pelvic floor for the actual birth of your baby. It plays an important role in keeping our pelvis in the correct skeletal orientation, along with right pressure on your nerves and ligaments. More so, a strong pelvic floor means that your baby is more likely to be in **the correct position for birth and your pelvis is more able to adjust easily** to allow your baby to pass through the pelvis and down to meet you faster and with more comfort.

It may seem counter intuitive to say we need to **relax** not tighten our pelvic floor muscles when we are birthing, as we have been working so hard at strengthening them. However, we know that tightening in any sense is not beneficial in birth, as relaxation for our whole body is what is required. If we do tighten the pelvic floor and when we birth our baby, it will reduce the space for our baby to born and may lead to an assisted delivery.

> *Some people are incorrectly advised to stop doing pelvic floor exercises before birth, so they don't have a 'too tight pelvic floor' when birthing. A strong pelvic floor is not a tight one - they are not the same thing! The problem can arise if a mother with a strong pelvic floor activity tightens her pelvic floor (not relaxes it) during birth, as with 'forced pushing' and this can lead to a longer and more difficult delivery.*

Remember 'smile for your sphincter?'

The vagina is also a sphincter, and it needs the right conditions to fully open and allow your baby to pass out easily. This is another reason why relaxation, a sense of calm and privacy while birthing is important. There is also a link between your open throat and your open vagina.

Open throat = open vagina

Open throat = relaxed pelvic floor

Say 'Arrhhh' or 'Who' As You Breathe Out

Quick Exercise:

1. Take a quick breath in through your nose and then on the out breathe say *'Arrhhhh'*. Repeat, but now become tense.
2. Take a quick breath in through your nose and then breathe out *'who'*. Only place your mouth in the right position to say 'who' (we only breathe, not say 'who'). It is like breathing on a feather or making a candle flicker. Repeat, but now become tense.

Which did you find most helpful? What was easier to stay relaxed?

'Arrhhh' pros and cons

- Easy to keep your lips and mouth loose.
- Need to remember to keep your jaw and neck relaxed.
- Good if you prefer sound when birthing.

'Who' pros and cons

- Easy to keep your jaw and neck relaxed.
- Need to remember to keep your lips and mouth loose.
- Good for those who prefer to be quiet in birthing.

The choice of how you breathe out is yours. So practice both and you know which one you may feel most comfortable with, and use on the day of your birth.

Key points to successful birth breathing (without the forced pushing)

- Wait for your 'urge'.
- Follow your body's lead.
- Relax your pelvic floor muscles.
- Open your mouth and your throat.
- Take a quick 'power breath'.
- Breathe out *'Arrrhhh'* (relax jaw and neck).

or

- Breathe out, *'Who'* gently blowing on a candle so it flickers.
- Be in an upright birthing position.
- Prepared your body through exercise.
- Have developed strong pelvic floor muscles.
- Your baby is in a good birthing position.

Birth breathing technique

You are almost there, and now your baby has started the journey down to your vagina and you start to feel your 'urge.' Your focus should be on listening to your body, following your 'birth breathing' and going with the sensations - your body will do the rest. **The breathing is purely to assist your body to birth your baby, but not 'pushing.'**

1. Birth Breathe only when in a Surge (contraction).
2. Take a quick power *breath in* through your nose, quickly collecting all the oxygen for a long out breath.
3. *Breathe in* 1,2, and *breathe out* 1,2,3,4,5,6,7,8,9,10. *(The count isn't important although may help you understand the length to breath).*
4. On the out breath, breathe out *'Arrrhhh'' or 'Who'.*
5. On the out breath, direct your breath downwards and forwards to your vagina.
6. Relax and release your pelvic floor and bowel muscles at all times.
7. Be directed by your body just how much assistance to provide.
8. Be fully relaxed. Your mouth and jaw should be soft with lips slightly open.
9. Repeat Birth Breathing as many times as needed for the duration of the surge.

Follow the lead of your baby and your body for a gradual decent (not staff prompts) and continue for each surge until crowning (baby's head at your rim of vagina).

Tip: *Practice Birth breathing after thirty-five weeks when you are doing a bowel movement. You will be relaxing and releasing these muscles during birthing. It will also enable you to practice relaxing the pelvic floor muscles. You will be surprised just how easy your bowel movements will become!*

At crowning, follow your Midwife/Obstetrician

When you have effectively breathed your baby down to crowning *(at the perineum)*, your baby's birth is almost over. Yet, it is vital to listen to your caregiver who will assist you in keeping your perineum intact and have no tearing.

Once your baby is resting on your perineum, your caregiver will often ask you to 'blow or pant.' The reasoning behind this is to slow down your delivery and allow your perineum all the time it needs to gradually unfold the layers of skin and muscles. The perineum can then stretch and allow the baby's head to pass through.

Just for a moment, try pushing, blowing or panting at the same time. It is difficult! Panting/blowing is simply a signal to slow down until the caregiver directs you to birth your baby again. Once your skin has stretched, it is just one small birth breath to deliver the head. Again, your caregiver will let you know when it is time. He or she is waiting for the baby's head to turn, and when this happens, the whole body turns which allows the shoulders to come out one at a time. Then the rest of the body easily follows.

Your perineum is able to stretch more than any other part of your body. It is perfectly designed to remain intact in birthing. Your perineal massage will further prepare your body for birthing.

PERFECT PUSHING (FOR INTERVENTION)

We all aim for natural, intervention-free birth. For most of us in hypnobirthing, that's exactly what we will get. At times intervention may be necessary to have a healthy mother and baby. As such, we need to understand the best way to birth our baby into the world. We know we won't get the natural 'urge' to birth our baby, so then our body can't birth our baby for us - We need to give it our best possible assistance.

If you are in this situation and following this perfect pushing, you are less likely to need further intervention. You are highly likely to birth your baby feeling relaxed and positive.

Big babies, posterior babies, poor positions

You could be concerned over having a very big baby, or perhaps your baby is not in the optimal position for birth. It could also be you are birthing in a more reclined position. You may find that learning the perfect pushing (*intervention*) could be helpful. Many natural birth mothers have avoided medical intervention by assisting their body to birth their baby with this technique.

Perfect pushing (intervention) technique

It is important to know the right muscles to tighten and relax while actively pushing your baby out. Here, we focus on using only the muscles you will need, and making sure all others stay relaxed. With this technique, your shoulders, neck and face will all stay perfectly relaxed. Being so, you will easily be able to continue your sense of calm and peace.

This technique will give you all the muscle power you need to actively push your baby out quickly and effectively. Equally important, by **relaxing the pelvic muscles,** you are creating a resistance-free path for your baby to birth easier.

By following this technique, there is much less likelihood of vacuum delivery (*ventouse*) or forceps and tearing. The baby will also benefit and received the full amount of oxygen and as result will unlikely become 'stuck' or distressed.

1. Start only when in a surge. If you don't know if you are in a surge, follow staff prompts.
2. Take a quick power *breath in* through your nose, quickly collecting all the oxygen for a long out breath.
3. *Breathe in* 1, 2 - <u>*tighten the top of your abdomen only.*</u>
4. *Breathe out* 1,2,3,4,5,6,7,8,9,10 – <u>*push down firmly*</u> with the top abdomen muscles (*similar to pushing down on plunger coffee*).
5. On the out breath, breathe out *'Arrrhhh' or 'Who.'* Don't hold your breath while pushing!).
6. On the out breath, direct your breath downwards and forward to your vagina.
7. Relax and release your pelvic floor muscles at all times. This is extremely important to do.
8. Be fully relaxed. Your mouth and jaw should be soft with lips slightly open.
9. Only push from your top abdomen area. This is vital to be free of tension elsewhere.
10. Repeat as many times as needed for the duration of the surge.

Tighten the top of your abdomen as hard as you can. Then push the top of the tightened abdomen downwards. It is important to keep your pelvic floor muscles relaxed!

When we are having a flow of urine, our pelvic floor is relaxed. Next time, at the end of your flow of urine, practice a few perfect pushing (intervention) to feel how relaxed your pelvic floor should be when birthing.

HYPNOBIRTHING BREATHING EXERCISES

In addition to the Hypnobirthing Home Study Course breathing techniques, it is useful for your birthing partners to be aware of your normal breathing patterns. In this way, they can recognize any changes to those patterns during the birthing time. Such changes could indicate rises in adrenalin or tension, and partners can help you through it.

1. Breathing exercise – Surge breathing

Get yourself in a comfortable position and turn off all distractions. If you are with your birth partner, ask him or her to sit with their back resting against a wall and with the knees apart, forming a contour chair for you to relax into. Sit between the knees, resting back against the chest. Your partner's arms are around you and the hands gently rested on your tummy, with the fingers facing down to your pelvis. He or she will need to pay particular attention to the feeling of your tummy rising and falling, being aware of the pace of your surge breathing.

Mother: Lie back and relax into your partner's arms. Close your eyes and begin surge breathing. With each breath in, think of sending your breath way down into your lower tummy to where your baby lies. Imagine the muscles of your abdomen are extremely relaxed. Listen to the sound of your breathing, keeping it calm, steady and rhythmical.

After a few minutes discuss with each other:

- What did you notice about the pace of your breathing?
- How did it differ from your partner?
- Did you naturally get in-sync, or were your breathing rates very different?

2. Breathing exercise - matching and pacing Surge breathing

Partners: During the birthing time, one of the key things to be looking out for is if there is any change in her Surge Breathing patterns. This can indicate a degree of anxiety, tension or fear. If this were to happen, one of the quickest and most effective ways to help her relax is to **slow down and exaggerate your own breathing pattern so that she will naturally get back in-sync with you.**

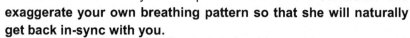

Mother: Sitting in the same position as before and begins surge breathing.

Partner: Sitting in the same position; concentrate on matching your breathing to hers. This can be a little strange and feel a bit forced, as pregnant women tend to breathe more slowly.

Once you are both in the same rhythm, it is important for the birth partner to keep this rhythm throughout the exercise.

Mother: After a short while, <u>consciously change</u> your breathing to a shallower, faster pace. Keep this up as long as possible, until you really have had enough and want to get back to your relaxed Surge Breathing.

Partner: Once you notice the change in her breathing, exaggerate your slow, deep breathing with the aim of encouraging her to go back to the surge breathing.

After a few minutes, discuss with each other:

- How did it feel when you were in-sync?
- How did it feel when you were not in-sync?
- Was it easy to keep breathing fast?
- How long did it last?
- How did it feel when returned to breathing together?

At the Birth: If the partner notices that the mother's breathing has become faster and shallower, then simply breathing loud, slow, deep breaths. This will remind her, in a non-verbal way, to get back into a quiet, deep rhythm.

It is worthwhile to practice this exercise of creating **synchronicity in Surge breathing** often. So that when the birth comes, it is second nature for your birth partner to assist your breathing.   Some mothers, when having a surge, prefer to be on their own and have their partners to just nearby. Do what works for you on the day. Your instincts will guide you.

3.   Breathing exercise - horse breathing

This may sound a bit odd, but it is a great exercise to help loosen and relax all the muscles in the jaw. This, in turn, will relax the muscles in the birth canal and perineum. Allow your lips to become really loose and floppy, then blow air out, making your lips gently vibrate. In general, this will naturally relax your jaw and neck and release tension. We often naturally do this when we feel relieved or want to relax. It is useful to remember to do this at intervals during the birth, especially as your baby is close to being born.

> In 1652, Philip Barrough wrote in his book 'The Method of Physick' that women were encouraged to breathe and relax their pelvic region, and that it eased the discomfort of birth.

 # BREATHING ESSENTIAL FOR BIRTH SUMMARY

Relaxation is the key to the hypnobirthing program. The more you can relax, the shorter and easier your birth will be.

Relaxation breathing

This breathing is simply to induce a sense of calm and relaxation. It is ideal in *pregnancy, the very early labor stages, and in between surges*. Relaxation breathing will instantly bring you to a relaxed state indeed.

Relaxation breathing is breathing for 1,2,3,4 and out 1,2,3,4,5,6,7,8

Surge breathing

This breathing is ideal when you are in *established birthing* for each surge *(contraction)*. By breathing in this unique way, it reduces any strong sensations to a very manageable level.

This breathing also makes each surge more effect to thin and open your cervix, so you can actually reduce your labor time.

Surge breathing is abdominal breathing - Slowly *breathe in,* for as long as you can to reach a comfortable number perhaps 10 and slowly *breathe out* for the same count.

Birth breathing

It is useful when you are actually *birthing* your baby and responding to your 'urge.' By working effectively with your body, your baby's entrance into the world is a safe, natural, easy, calm, comfortable and an enjoyable experience.

Birth Breathing is a quick breath in and long breath out, while relaxing your body and responding to it effectively.

VISUALIZE YOUR AMAZING BIRTH

The mind is an incredibly powerful tool, through which you can use imagery and visualization to help reduce stress and sensations, as well as to increase health and wellbeing.

Using visualization as part of your birth preparation helps to take you into a deeply relaxed state, which naturally helps to reduce levels of discomfort by 'switching off' from what may be happening in your body. By practicing visualization during your pregnancy, it will become second nature and very comforting. Once mastered, your mind is already familiar with the process during the birth.

It is important to reiterate that just because we use the words "visual" it does not mean that you have to be able to "see" pictures. Many people find it difficult to visualize and may shy away from following this technique. It does not matter how you do it - the process is more important!

Some people simply hear sounds or feel the experience of being there. That is perfectly fine and right for you. Whatever sense you use the most, and no matter how you experience the world, just go with 'visualising' whatever way feels right for you. However, for the sake of simplicity, we will continue to use the word "visualization."

 "The soul never thinks without a picture." - Aristotle

Visualization success in many fields

We have studied the intricate and amazing power of the mind. We have also learned how emotions, particularly unhelpful ones like fear, can specifically interrupt the body and the natural birth process. The good news is: positive thoughts, emotions, relaxation and visualization can help the body and enhance its ability to birth freely and effectively. That is, after all what hypnobirthing is about.

It was first recorded that the Grecians used deep relaxation and visualization as the main treatment in freeing people from illness. For centuries, tribal customs across the globe use superstitions to bring about physical and emotional healing. It is only now in the last few decades are we beginning to increase our awareness and acceptance of the ways in which self-hypnosis can physiologically affect our cellular level and mentally reprogram behaviours and beliefs which are blocking our success.

Have a look next time you are watching the Olympics or other important sporting events. Watch the athletes mentally rehearsing their performance just prior to the event. With such high competition stakes, most athletes will:

1.   Perform relaxation breathing.
2.   Self-hypnotize to block out noise, distractions and provide focus.

3.   Use a confidence trigger (*similar to our relaxation trigger*).
4.   Quickly visualize themselves performing at the highest level.

Being in a relaxed state, feeling good, focused, and visualising their win; now these athletes are ready to perform at their best. This success formula is also being used in the medicine and the business world to enable people to perform at the highest possible level.

What exactly is visualization?

Visualization is the process of mentally producing pictures, or playing a movie in your head and directing your thoughts to a specific outcome. Imagining your wonderful birth with everything going the way you planned and feeling the joyful emotion, is an example of an effective visualization.

Daydreaming is a simple example of visualization. Yet here, you often just allow your mind to wander aimlessly without specific action. You are being led by your thoughts rather than specifically and consciously choosing to direct your 'own movie.'

During **self-hypnosis**, the brain and nervous system are saturated with a picture of a specific, sensory vision that seems so real. It then becomes imprinted in the brain. This occurs exactly the same way real experiences become stored within the memory of the subconscious. When a person is in a relaxed state, like hypnosis, the mind more easily accepts the imagery and suggested vision as 'real.' If we visualize continually the same image or scene over again, this tips our belief scales and has the desired outcome.

Now back to you

Your mind stores all your experiences and memories and then holds them until they are needed as references again in the future. By giving your mind a new set of wonderful birthing experiences and responses, when the time comes to birth, these are triggered in your mind and you automatically follow the new set of responses. Clinical trials have proven the success of giving these types of suggestions when in hypnosis.[16]

Remember, your inner mind does not know the difference between things that you have imagined and things that are real.

*"Experimental and clinical psychologists have proven beyond a shadow of a doubt that the human nervous system cannot tell the difference between an 'actual' experience and an experience imagined vividly in detail".[1] - **Dr. Maltz***

As we discussed in Unit 2, you have the same physiological response to pretend or imagined danger, such as a horror film, as you have to real danger. Watching a horror film is not real although the image that is imprinted in your mind is real and your body kicks off an adrenalin response. We know the negative impact that adrenaline has on birth, yet just imagine the benefits and potential if we used visualization in a positive way.

By creating your own "Amazing Birth Films" showing the positive birth outcomes, you are more likely to get the same response when the 'film' becomes the reality of your birthing day.

---

[16] Alman, B. M. & Carney, R. E., "Consequences of Direct and Indirect Suggestion on Success of Post-Hypnotic Behaviour", American Journal of Clinical Hypnosis, Vol. 23 1080.

How visualization influences memory

Some experts suggest that memory is a process of reconstruction, rather than a recall of established events. This memory reconstruction comes from stored components involving elaborations, distortions, and omissions. Every time we remember an event, it is merely a recall of the last reconstruction of the experience. Our memory of situations or experiences in our lives will change a little, and this happens each time we bring a memory to our minds. Perhaps the memory has more vivid happy emotions with the sun a little brighter, the weather just right, and little details changed or lost. This difference in memory may help to explain why two people experiencing the same situation have very different recollections of the same event.

As memories are more fluid than a fixed recall of events, we naturally change our memories and past experiences. Youngston studied 'déjà vu' and proposed it is when we are in a relaxed state, daydreaming or visualising a possible future. Such as great birth experience (*or one filled with intervention*), we will often find ourselves with a sense of recognition (*déjà vu*) and occurs when we are achieving a good 'match' between the present experience and our stored data of the birth event.[17]

*"**Déjà vu**, from French, literally "already seen," is the phenomenon of having the strong sensation that an event or experience currently being experienced has been experienced in the past, whether it has actually happened or not". **Wikipedia 2013***

The same is true for 'memories' you want to influence for the future. Why not use this phenomenon of the **flexibility of your memory** to create your best possible birth experience. The aim in your visualization session is to make the birthing experience in your mind **as real as possible** for you. In that way, the mind is more likely to accept the images as 'real' and keep it stored. Then later when you do birth, your inner mind recalls these images as a type of **birth blue print**, for what to follow and creates a sense of familiarity - that it has been here before.

Guided imagery and visualization

For most people, there is a wonderful sense of relaxation and letting go during a hypnosis session. Many people do experience a feeling of sinking or going down, so we often use the word 'deepening' to explain this feeling.

In the Hypnobirthing Home Study Course recordings, we frequently use guided imagery. It is, after all, an easy and wonderful way of encouraging your mind to step away from "reality" and into your own world of imagination. This visualization increases your sense of focus and heightened awareness, and it helps you connect with the inner part of yourself. In addition, it encourages and directs your mind to focus on helpful birth images and experiences.

Create your 'special place'

When you are in a surge (*contraction*) and practicing your Surge breathing, begin by thinking about a special place. This can be any place you have been to that you have really loved: maybe somewhere on holiday, a garden, the mountains or even your own room. Think of any location or setting which represents a feeling of calm, relaxation, happiness or peace. Go there in your imagination when you are birthing your baby. You can even make it up or go somewhere you have seen on the TV. For me, my 'special place' is on a Caribbean island, with warm gentle waves and white, soft sand. It is a wonderful safe haven, a sanctuary to go to where I know that other thoughts will not reach me, and where I will always have a deep sense of happiness and calm.

---

[17] Youngson, R. "Deja Vu". The Royal Society of Medicine Health Encyclopaedia. Dr R.M. Youngson. Retrieved 1 October 2012.

Be creative! Your imagination is limitless. Whatever you choose to visualize or imagine, make your experience as detailed as possible: see it, smell it, taste it, touch it, hear it, and, lastly, throw in a dose of emotion - love it, cherish it, enjoy it and marvel at it!

"Your subconscious mind recognizes and acts upon only thoughts which have been well-mixed with emotion or feeling; and, you will get no appreciable results until you learn to reach your subconscious mind with thoughts or spoken words which have been well emotionalized with belief." - Napoleon Hill

A study by Edmund Jacobson showed that visualising an activity produced a measurable reaction in the muscles. Likewise, by performing a mental rehearsal of how you would like your birth to play out, you are actually implanting a learned memory of an already successful birth. You are also informing your inner mind of what you expect it to achieve.

People can beat a lie detector by repeatedly visualising, feeling and fully experiencing a 'new truth' until they confidently believe the 'new truth' is actually a reality.

Visualization - the head down position

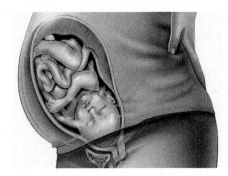

We know how there is strong connection between our minds and our bodies. Therefore, we make use of this connection when visualising the optimal position that our baby needs to be in. In this way, we are one step closer to having the natural birth that we are entitled to have.

Please put this picture in a place where you will see it every day.

Visualization - your perineum gently opening

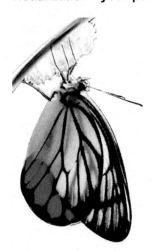

You can't hurry the development of the butterfly in the chrysalises. We wouldn't dream of pulling this cocoon apart to help the butterfly emerge, as we trust that nature knows the best time and way to develop and bring into the world a beautiful butterfly.

The same is true about your birth. Trust in nature and your body to perfectly develop and birth your baby at the right time. When this wonderful birthing day arrives and your baby's head is resting on your perineum, remember to slow down your delivery until all the skin and muscles of the perineum gradually stretch and open fully to easily allow your baby to emerge while you deliver in comfort and ease.

Please put this picture in a place where you will see it every day.

DEEP RELAXATION TECHNIQUES FOR BIRTH

Relaxation sounds easy, but in fact it is something that needs practice in order to achieve the kind of deep relaxation needed for your birth. An untrained mother to be would find it very hard, if not impossible, to suddenly relax during her birthing time. Often it is said, "try to relax" and the mother bravely "tries." She then makes her body appear still and quiet. But that is very different from genuinely letting go of all the tension in her body.

Relaxation is your foundation. Everything else depends on it and everything builds on it. If you are tense during a surge, the uterus has to work twice as hard to do the same amount of work, as the other muscles are straining against the uterus, making the sensations much stronger.

Learning how to relax at will is a skill

The purpose of relaxation is to ensure your body stays totally limp, thereby, allowing your birthing muscles to work unimpeded by other bodily tensions. This may sound easy. Truth is, it is simple but not that easy! Initially it may take all your concentration to keep your whole body limp and free of tension. **Your ability to relax during surges will directly correlate to your degree of comfort**.

To become skillful at relaxing, you have to become efficient at noticing tension and then releasing it. Then once you recognize it, you can release it. Relaxation is not like going to sleep where you just wait for your body to relax. Truth is relaxation is something that you do with intention.

Relaxation is something you can do yourself

You will be amazed at how often we hold tension in our body. Find out for yourself!

As you go about your daily routine, check to see if there is any tension in your body. Drop your shoulders, relax your hands, and relax your back. If you feel any tension rising in your body, take a deep breath, a long exhale (*one relaxation breath*) and actively relax that part of your body. By doing this several times a day, you will soon recognize when your body feels tense and when it is relaxed.

Make your own relaxation session

Listening to a Hypnobirthing relaxation track is such a wonderful way of learning relaxation. You will learn that the more you do it, the easier it becomes. Unlike learning other new skills, it is wonderfully enjoyable and relaxing from the outset. It is simply a matter of lying back, closing your eyes and finding peace and calm in your body. There are many different techniques for achieving a relaxed state and many different types of visualizations which help you achieve this. Alternatively, why not create your own relaxation with these techniques:

1.   Fractional relaxation

One popular method is a '*fractional relaxation.*' This involves focusing on different parts of your body and gradually releasing tension in each area. You can use colours to show a change from tension to relaxation as you start at the top of your head and gradually move down to your face, your neck, your shoulders, your back and so on. This is especially useful if you are experiencing discomfort in any part of your body, such as your pelvis or back. As you can linger on that area, imagine that you are releasing all discomfort, filling that area with warmth, comfort and a sense of calm.

As you move down across your stomach, you can spend some time focusing on your baby. Imagine your baby smiling and moving freely, seeing your baby in your imagination. You are becoming calm and may experience a feeling of heaviness, lightness or tingling. This is perfectly normal, and it is a sign that your body is really relaxing and letting go.

2. Progression through counting

A second and very powerful way of relaxing the body is using a form of *'progression through counting or a sense of movement.'* You may like to imagine that you are at the top of a safe, wide staircase with a firm handrail and eight steps ahead of you. Imagine that as you slowly and carefully go down each step, you become more and more relaxed, letting all your muscles become more and more limp, soft and at ease. As you count down each step, your body becomes progressively heavier, softer and more relaxed. By the time you get to one, you are fully relaxed and at ease.

RELAXATION TRIGGERS

1,2,3,4 ... Relax

A relaxation trigger is a powerful and effective way to instantly feel relaxed by actively creating a **trigger and response event**.

Every action has a reaction, many of which are instinctive. For example, if you feel heat or pain, you instantly move your hand away. As you hear your name, you answer. If you hear a siren while driving, you suddenly focus your attention to your driving. If you see a red light, you stop. Pavlov was the first to formally recognize the trigger and response by noticing his dogs salivating on the anticipation of food. In the same way, it is easy to **create a relaxation response to specific trigger**. This will enable you to instantly create sense of relaxation and calm when you are birthing your baby.

Embedding the Relax 1,2,3,4 technique

Throughout the Hypnobirthing Home Study Course recordings, you will hear the phrases again and again

'.... takes you to an even deeper level of relaxation and calm. Feeling, being even more relaxed. 1,2,3,4 ..... relax. And the more you practice the easier it is to take yourself into wonderful deep relaxation. 1,2,3,4.....relax.

The purpose of this statement, is to create a sense of relaxation every time you hear or say the phrase *'1,2,3,4....relax.'* The more that you hear this and are already in a relaxed state, the stronger the association will become. If you need a little extra sense of relaxation at the birth, all need to do is say to yourself *'1,2,3,4....relax'* and your body will respond accordingly.

You can do this yourself, instead of listening to the recording; by simply repeating those phrases to yourself or have your partner say those to you.

However, it is important to remember that you need to **do this over and over again**. When you get a new ringtone on your mobile phone, in the beginning you often ignore it, as you don't think it's your phone. However over time you remember, as you have made the subconscious association and soon you automatically reach for it when it rings.

1,2,3,4 ....Relax and your birth partner's touch

You can deepen your relaxation by creating an even **more powerful relaxation trigger**. You can tell your subconscious that every time you feel your **partner's hand on your shoulder** (*trigger*), your body will respond by becoming wonderfully **relaxed and calm** (*response*). The more you do this, the more this new response is embedded, and the more your subconscious accepts this new pattern or way of doing things.

Shoulder (trigger) ⟹ **relaxed and calm (response)**

Partner: Stand next to the mother to be, and in a calm gentle manner slowly say '1,2,3,4.....Relax', as you say the word 'relax' place your hand on her shoulder for a few seconds.

Mother: As the hand is placed on your shoulder, consciously feel your body in a deep state of relaxation.

Tip: You can also create your own relaxation trigger by putting your own hand on your

Birth music relaxation trigger

Another great way of achieving a learned triggered response is through music. By listening to the same relaxing birth music every time you practice your own relaxation and breathing exercises, you are making a subconscious association with that music and deep relaxation. Therefore, when you play that music during the birth, it is yet another way for the birthing brain and body to work together to stay deeply calm and relaxed.

TOUCH RELAXATION TRIGGER

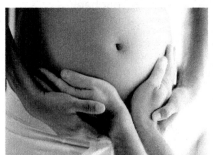

Another technique that can significantly aid in developing your skill at relaxation is one that involves touch. During touch relaxation, your partner places his or her hand on your tensed muscles. In response, you relax your muscles toward his or her hand. Practicing this form of nonverbal communication will help you learn to respond with complete relaxation to your partner's touching, stroking, and massaging during labor.

After a while, verbal cues won't be necessary at that time your muscles will be conditioned to relax automatically in response to your partner's touch. As soon as you feel your partner's touch, begin to consciously release the muscles to be relaxed as possible. Touch relaxation is one of the best techniques to use during your birthing time. Although this technique is meant to be done with the aid of a partner, after performing it several times, many women find they can take themselves to a very relaxed place on their own.

Following the steps of this guide will help your entire body reach a state of complete relaxation. All cues to be given slowly, calmly and lovingly. This type of massage is best conducted with **Relaxation Breathing** as the mother has already learnt this type of relaxation. The partner reads the verbal cues and on the mother's long out breath, puts the hands on the appropriate area for relaxation.

Strengthening the 1,2,3,4....relax trigger

At many times during the touch relaxation, you will be asked to 'touch to the mother's shoulder'. With the mother being in such a relaxed state, you are automatically increasing the effects of relaxation and strengthening the 1,2,3,4 ... relax trigger.

*When performing this relaxation, put your choice of **Birth Music** on in the background. It will 'anchor' in a relaxation response when practicing at home. When you are at your birthing time, you will find it easier to relax.*

Touch relaxation technique

Partner's verbal cues to Mother	Partner's touch response
1	"Close your eyes, and start your **Relaxation Breathing** – in, 1,2,3,4 and out 1,2,3,4,5,6,7,8. Continue with this breathing now and for the whole relaxation. Begin to let the tension flow from your body (*pause*). Release any tightness in your **head** starting at the top of your head, and then moving down your sides and back of your head."	Place hands on sides of **head** near temples. Feel the forehead relax.
2	"Lower your **eyebrows**. Just let them drop"	Place hands on **eyebrows**. Feel the eyebrows relax.
3	"Close your **eyes**. Feel your eyelids becoming heavy, your eyes sinking back into your head."	Place hands *gently* on **eyelids**. Observe relaxation
4	"Let your **jaw** drop. Part your lips slightly."	Place hands on sides of **jaw.** Feel the jaw drop.
5	"Allow your **head** to rest against the pillow, (If her head is not supported, say: "slightly lower your chin.")	Hold the top of her **head** gently. Observe relaxation.
6	"Feel your **shoulder** blades open outward and downward"	Rest hands on front of **shoulders.** Observe relaxation of upper body.
7	"Starting at your **right shoulder** move any tightness down your upper arm (*pause*) past your elbow (*pause*) down your lower arm (*pause*) past your wrist (*pause*) through your hand (*pause*) and out your fingers."	**Touch in sequence**, right shoulder to elbow, to lower arm to wrist, hands and fingers. Observe relaxation.
8	"Starting at your **left shoulder,** move any tightness down your upper arm (*pause*) past your elbow (*pause*) down your lower arm (*pause*) past your wrist (*pause*) through your hand (*pause*) and out your fingers."	**Touch in sequence**, left shoulder to elbow, to lower arm to wrist, hands and fingers. Observe relaxation.
9	"Concentrate on your **breathing.** Slowly breathe in oxygen through your nose and send it to your baby 1,2,3,4; slowly exhale 1,2,3,4,5,6,7,8, releasing tension. With each out breath release a little more tension."	**Observe relaxation**
10	"Remember to continue with your **Relaxation Breathing**. Breathe in again, 1,2,3,4 and a long breath out ...right down your back, starting at the base of your neck, and slowly moving down your upper back, past your ribs, down into your waist and into your hips. With each out breath release a little more tension."	**In sequence** place hand on back on neck, upper back and lower back and then hips.
11	"Breathe and relax right down (*pause*) starting at your **right hip**, move any tightness down your thigh (*pause*) past your knee (*pause*) down your calf (*pause*) past your ankle (*pause*) through your foot (*pause*) and out your toes."	**In sequence** place hand on **RIGHT** hip, thigh, knee, calf, ankle, foot and toes.
12	"Breathe and relax right down (*pause*) starting at your **left hip,** move any tightness down your thigh (*pause*) past your knee (*pause*) down your calf (*pause*) past your ankle (*pause*) through your foot (*pause*) and out your toes."	**In sequence** place hand on **LEFT** hip, thigh, knee, calf, ankle, foot and toes.
13	"Feel **every limb** become heavy, your feet (*pause*) lower legs (*pause*) thighs (*pause*) hips, (*pause*) hands, (*pause*) arms, (*pause*) shoulders."	Gentle touch both **shoulders** when spoken.

14	'Feel the force of gravity pulling you **down** and into the earth *(pause)* you are sinking, sinking down."	Touch both **shoulders.**
15	"Your **knees** feel very heavy. Let them flop apart to the sides."	Touch both **knees.**
16	"Feel your **whole body** melting and spreading across the floor *(pause)*. Feel the sensation of tension flowing outward."	Touch both **shoulders.**
17	"Now take a moment to go over your body. Is there any area still holding **tension**? If so, think about bringing some heat to that area *(pause)*. Feel the warmth of the sun bringing relaxation."	Touch both **shoulders.**
18	'1,2,3,4 *(pause)* **Relax**'. Your whole body is now wonderfully relaxed and your mind is at ease.'	Touch both **shoulders.**
19	'When you are ready, open your eyes *(pause)* and gradually come back to the room."	-

 You can combine all these triggers so that your partner can string them together to take you into a deeply relaxed state, quickly and easily.

MATERNITY OPTIONS AND CHOICES

For many, choosing to become pregnant was a decision that took some time to make. Most couples have to talk through careful considerations and weighing up a number of factors to welcome a child into your life at just the right time.

Now you may think the major decisions have finished! In fact, they are just starting. And one of the most important choices that you will make in having your wonderful natural birth is your maternity care provider. Who do you see? Where do you go for your care? How do you find out what is available out there? And most important of all, what is the best form of care right for you?

When a woman is pregnant for the first time, it can be a daunting and a confusing process to discover what maternity care options are available. Often the first step is the GP, who as an individual has their own preferences in birthing. Some women do feel pressured at this time to follow the advice of their GP, as they willingly do for sickness.

Yet, pregnancy is a natural a normal bodily process. There's an increasing variety of pregnancy and birth options for women to choose from. However, some women like those who live in rural and remote areas, there may be little choice. Many women talk to their friends to get information and this can be a great way to get an inside view of what is available. But remember, it's someone else's view and it's influenced by an individual experience, so start now to look at all the options available to you at this time. Then make your own informed choice!

To gain a better insight into what you may actually wish for your birth, you need to willingly let go of ingrained fears and beliefs about what actually is the best and safest option for you and your baby. It is vital that you weigh up all the information carefully and make a decision based on what birth you truly feel is the best option for you.

Are you making your choices based on other's views, your fear of the unknown or other incongruent beliefs? Ensure your choice brings you peace, fulfillment and happiness.

Brazil has the world's highest caesarean rate of 49% compared to 13% in the Netherlands.

Mother's Thoughts

"I didn't really know where to go and who to have care for us and it was harder than I would have thought. The GP who did my pregnancy test said, 'Do you have private health insurance that covers maternity?' And as I did, he gave me the name of someone he said was a good obstetrician and he knew him from university days. It was only after going to the obstetrician and realising I didn't like his manner and attitude to my questions that I started to ask around. It was then a friend told me about birth centres and midwives and that there were other options.

I don't think it should be like that, there needs to be more independent information. I was about 30 weeks pregnant and I wanted to change from my obstetrician. One mum I met said she loved hers because she didn't even need to prepare for the birth. She seemed really pleased that he made all the decisions and enjoyed handing over full control. Well, that didn't sit right with me. This is my baby and I want to birth naturally, my way. Another obstetrician proudly said he had a 70% caesarean rate and loved surgery and if it was up to him, he would do a caesarean on everyone at 38 weeks. He said, 'just think of that, you could plan the date of your birth with no contractions or uncertainly, just brilliant!' No thanks!

I investigated a midwife lead birthing centre, but as they are so popular, I couldn't get in. I bravely investigated a home birth. It scared me to death thinking about it! It was total 360 degree turn around from where I started. My friends looked horrified when I told them about the home birth. They thought it was like performing surgery on my kitchen bench!

I took a deep breath and saw an independent midwife to ask questions. After speaking with Janet, she made such a difference and I started to feel confident about the birth at home. I did lots and lots of research!! I discovered that in uncomplicated births, there is no extra risk than a hospital birth. I took the plunge and planned to birth at home. First of all, I put on the 'Release the Fear of Birth' track about 100 times to get me confident about the birth! But I did it and I am so proud. It was just my fear of anything going wrong that lead me down to the obstetrician route. Once I was brave enough to stop, pause and assess what I did want; then it was just the fear and peer pressure from others that were stopping from having the most anointed, peaceful and beyond words birth experience.

Katelyn was born three weeks ago, at 41 weeks and 5 days, after an 11 hour easy labor. It was long, but worth every minute of it as I was able to use all the hypnobirthing techniques. This birth was the most mesmerising, cherished and blessed experience of my life (until my next birth of course!). I know it wouldn't have been like that if I had been in a hospital. My advice to you girls is - take a good long hard look at with who and where you plan to birth and make sure it is what you want rather than being ruled by fear or others. Lots of love to you all." **Joslin Jacobson, Perth Australia**

Maternity options around the world

We may know what is available to us in our own country, yet it is worthwhile taking a look at how births occur around the world with a modern birthing system. It may give you some insight into a different point of view and challenge your own thoughts and beliefs about birth. We will start the process off with the Australian maternity system and then make our way to our neighbors of New Zealand. We then go across the seas to the United States and United Kingdom, with a hop and jump over the pond to the Netherlands.

THE AUSTRALIAN MATERNITY SYSTEM

Public hospital care (74% of births) – Medicare: no cost

In Australia, most pregnant women, after obtaining a referral from their general practitioner (GP), birth at a public hospital. Depending on where they live and the hospital they choose, they may be able to access several different options.

- **Midwives Clinics.** Many major public hospitals have 'midwives antenatal clinics' that are run by midwives. These maternal health care providers are skilled professionals who are qualified to provide complete care for women experiencing normal pregnancy and childbirth. If any complications develop, the midwives refer women to doctors at the hospital. Midwives focus on more than the physical aspects of the pregnancy. They regard the emotional and psychosocial needs of women as a high priority. Different midwives will support at birth and most births will be attended by doctors. Women enjoy seeing the same midwife for their care during pregnancy as a trust and relationship develops.

- **Midwifery Group Practice.** This come usually as a small group of midwives who work together to provide full antenatal, labor, birth, and postnatal care to women. Doctors do not attend uncomplicated births, yet are at hand when needed. The effectiveness of continuity of midwifery care is largely due to the relationship of trust that is built up during the pregnancy, birth and postnatal periods. This form of care results in less intervention and higher long term breastfeeding rates, as well as lower rates of postnatal depression. Women experiencing this form of care have been shown to feel well prepared for labor, to perceive labor staff as caring, to feel in control during labor and feel well prepared for parenting.

- **General Practitioner Shared Care Programs (Small Cost).** Such set up is when pregnancy care is shared between a general practitioner and a hospital. This provides women with the convenient access of their antenatal care in their own local area. They also may have a good relationship with their general practitioner and want to continue this care in their pregnancy. Women will attend a local public hospital for the birth and some antenatal appointments with an obstetrician. This obstetrician may or not be the same one at the birth.

Birth Centre care (1% of births)

Australia will only accommodate women with very low risk pregnancies at a birth center, and these centres are mostly located in hospitals. Staffed and run by midwives, these centres provide medical back up should complications develop. If you have chosen an obstetrician for your care, ask them if they will attend your birth in a birth center as many will not.

Birth centres provide a home-like environment where midwives care for women throughout pregnancy. These health care givers also provide assistance to give birth as actively and naturally as possible. There is a great emphasis in birth centres on empowering women and helping them to feel in control of the whole experience.

Research exploring birth experiences and outcomes shows that women under the care of midwives through a birth center have lower intervention rates. They are also found more satisfied than with other forms of care. This is particularly so when midwives work in a team midwifery arrangement in birth centres where women experience even greater continuity of care. Book early, though, because birth centres are very popular and often over booked.

Private Hospital care (cost associated: 25% of births)

If you have the appropriate private health insurance (*or are uninsured and willing to pay*) you can choose a private obstetrician to provide your antenatal care. Obstetricians are doctors specializing in pregnancy and childbirth. These birthing health professionals will attend your birth in a private or public hospital.

Costs for private care are not completely covered by a health fund, so you will need to pay part of the fee. There are enormous variations in obstetricians and hospital's fees so explore this carefully. The average expenditures for this would be **$2,445 - $8,355** at the average. This is roughly including prenatal care, birth and post-natal care for those with full private health insurance.[18]

Home Birth care (cost associated: less than 1% of births)

In Australia, only a few hundred women each year choose to give birth at home. This option put these women under the care of mainly independent midwives during the birth. These midwives work for themselves rather than a hospital, with a cost of **$4000- $5000**. Some midwifery services will be covered by a Medicare and private health fund rebates. It's best to check ahead if your midwife is covered.

With this arrangement, the same midwife or small group of midwives provides pregnancy, birth and postnatal care. If you choose this option and complications occur during the pregnancy or birth, it may mean you will need to have your baby in hospital. Most midwives will accompany and support you when this occurs and continue to care for you along with the hospital doctors and midwives. Intervention rates in birth are low and women's satisfaction with care is extremely high when cared for by independent midwives.

Currently there are a couple of publicly funded (no cost) home birth programs run through the hospital system. Check to see if there is one in your local area.

THE NEW ZEALAND MATERNITY OPTIONS

The New Zealand model of maternity care is perhaps the most collaborative and integrative of the five countries here studied. In this model, a pregnant woman may to choose to receive care from a midwife, an FP/GP, an obstetrician, or a combination of providers. However, one person must be identified as the lead maternity care.

In most instances, maternity, birth and antenatal care is provided as part of the national health care, meaning little or no cost to birthing mothers. Options of home births, birth centres and hospitals are part of the birthing choices.

Interestingly, as women have wide choice of their care providers, some 78% of women in New Zealand select a midwife to provide all their pregnancy, birth and postnatal care. If complications arise, then obstetricians attend to such cases. However New Zealand has lower caesarean section rates than Australia and most of the world. Women can also have the choice to select a private obstetrician (*at cost*), yet this is a less popular option.

---

[18] Australia, NIB , 'The Cost of Having a Baby, Private Health Insurance' 2013

Your rights during pregnancy and birth[1]

In New Zealand, it is made clear to women of her birthing rights.

You have the right:

- *To be treated with dignity, cultural sensitivity and respect at all times.*
- *To choose your place of birth.*
- *To choose your caregiver/s, and to change your caregivers/s at any time.*
- *To choose who will be present at your birth and to ask others to leave.*
- *Before agreeing to any procedures or being given any drug, medication or test, to ask about any side effects or risks to yourself or your baby. You can accept or refuse any treatments.*
- *To choose how you will give birth and to feel free to follow your feelings and instincts during birth.*

THE UNITED KINGDOM MATERNITY OPTIONS

In the United Kingdom, midwifery is integral to maternity care where most midwives work for the National Health Service (NHS) and provide prenatal, birth, and postnatal care. To increase continuity of care, midwives have formed small teams among their fellows which provide complete care to a small number of women. Despite midwives' role in maternity care, all women have the option of choosing an OB/GYN as their lead medical provider by being referred by a midwife/GP.

The scope of practice for midwives in the United Kingdom is more extensive than other parts of the world and as such, these maternal care professionals undergo more training. Midwives provide prenatal care and many do ultrasounds as part of prenatal care, electronic foetal monitoring (EFM), prescribe analgesics, artificial oxytocin, cut and repair episiotomies, deliver breech babies, a few use vacuum extraction and forceps, and injections, all without consulting a doctor.

> (i) *It is rare to hire the services of a private obstetrician in the UK, as public health system fully covers maternity, birth and antenatal care. Importantly, private health insurance in the UK does not cover maternity and birth, so this influences choice.*

Home births, birth centres, and hospitals are all choices for birthing mothers, with a national home birth rate of around 2.4% Transfers from home to hospital during labor or just after birth are about 20% of mothers to be were transferred to hospital.

THE UNITED STATES MATERNITY OPTIONS

In the United States, the maternity care model is unique in that most of the care of pregnant women is provided by obstetricians (69%) and private general/family practitioners continue to provide more maternity care compared to other countries (22.4%). Midwives have traditionally played a less significant role, yet their influence is growing annually (7.65%).

The United States has a very limited safety net for health care, and that also includes maternity and birth services. In most instances, if you do not have private health insurance, there will be a large out of pocket expense. Most obstetricians have a global maternity fee, and that fee covers all of your office visits with the doctor as well as his or her presence at the delivery of your baby. This fee varies from practice to practice and from state to state, ranging from US**$2,500 to $5,000.** This global maternity fee applies whether you have insurance or not. If you don't have insurance, prenatal care, birth hospitalisation can run from US$10,000 to $100,000 or more.

While this dollar figure is dependent upon the type of delivery you have and where you deliver, the fees are still staggering. As the cost of health care on the rise, some new families are choosing to have home births or prefer to use a birthing center rather than a traditional hospital maternity ward. Typically, these alternative birth options have a set fee for prenatal care and delivery fees, effectively cutting down the total cost to deliver your new tiny bundle of joy.

NETHERLANDS MATERNITY OPTIONS

The Dutch attitude is that pregnancy is not an illness and that home births are the norm. Health insurance does not cover the cost of a hospital birth unless there was a real medical imperative. If you feel you need to see an obstetrician, you must go through your general practitioner and without a referral; you cannot even get an appointment.

> *"The Netherlands has the highest percentage of home births in the Western world,"* **Sjaak Toet,** The Chairman of the Dutch Association of Midwives KNOV

In the Netherlands, 30% of Dutch women birth at home and 60% birth in hospital, mostly for medical reasons. The 10% of Dutch women opt to deliver their babies in birth centres. While more than half of all Dutch women still end up in hospital, this is due to midwives hospitalizing if there is a low medical risk, and the 60% hospital figure includes women who started delivering at home, but were transferred when problems arose.

Midwife Thoughts

"It is a question of attitude: we are matter of fact. Women tell me, 'My mother had all her kids at home and that always went well. Why should I go to hospital?' Women usually say themselves, that giving birth at home is more relaxed because you don't have to rush to the hospital panting, give birth and be sent home again after a quick shower. If there's nothing wrong with you or your baby, you are not kept in hospital (overnight) in the Netherlands," **Sjaak Toet, Rotterdam, Netherlands**

 In Scandinavian countries, such as Sweden, midwives deliver most babies, and they have the lowest rates of babies dying in the world.

PRIVATE OBSTETRICIANS

Choosing an obstetrician can be a challenge to select the best doctor for you and your baby to give the birth that you wish for. As obstetricians are individuals just like us, there is a wide range of preferences in their delivery methods, intervention rates and attitudes to natural birthing. It is most important that you feel comfortable and fully at ease with your obstetrician and have synergy with your birth goals. Above all else, on the day of the birth, your objective is to be fully relaxed, and trusting of your caregivers is such a crucial part of the success of your birthing day.

Obstetricians are highly trained professionals whose expertise is ideally suited for high risk pregnancies and births. Here lies the benefit and also the downside in one. Obstetricians are ideal to have around if a complication arises (*benefit*). However, for healthy, low risk pregnancies and births, there are lower rates of interventions (*with similar safety ratings*) with midwife led prenatal care and birthing. Like any statistic, it doesn't account for individuals and just as no two pregnancies and births are the same, the same is true for your obstetrician.

If you are thinking about choosing this maternity care route, asking a series of questions can give you confidence in your choice.

Questions to ask an Obstetrician (before you commit)

What is your view on natural birth? *(Normal vaginal birth, with no intervention or drugs; ensure your definition is the same as your doctors.)*

- What is your view on hypnobirthing?
- Roughly, what proportion of women in your care gave birth without intervention and drugs?
- What is your caesarean rate and what are the main reasons for caesareans?
- What is your induction rate and what are the main reasons for inductions?
- What birthing positions would you support?

Asking obstetricians a number of questions is another good way to discover their position and action on instances where intervention is needed. Some obstetricians love surgery and perform best in high risk pregnancy and birthing situations. Others will actively encourage natural birth and allow you to 'run your own show,' only being there as a backup in case they are needed.

The more questions you ask early on, the more you will soon get a feeling of how well the two of you will work together during the pregnancy and birth. These questions are just the start and once you have worked out your birth plan (Unit 4), it is imperative that you have your obstetrician's full backing, knowing that your birthing wishes will be respected.

It is important that women also realise that private obstetricians usually come to the delivery ward close to the birth, just in time to get the gloves on! Midwives provide all the labor care and communicate on the phone with the obstetrician. If there are any complications or the birth is imminent, then they will call the obstetrician. Most likely, birthing women have not even met the midwife and have had a relationship with only the obstetrician. In the postnatal ward, midwives will also be the ones to care for you. Women who have chosen this route are willing to sacrifice the unfamiliarity with their allocated midwife, for the highly regarded obstetrician's expertise in case of a change of plans to the birthing is required.

 Mother's Thoughts

"I went down the obstetrician route. As a low risk pregnancy I knew that technically I didn't need to go down this way. But I did like the doctor and she was the one who actually encouraged me to do Hypnobirthing and told me what books to read. I connected with her and she patiently answered my questions including the weird and crazy hypothetical's from my husband. While she wouldn't do everything on my birth plan, we worked through some alternatives that made us both feel good with the planning of the birth. On the day of the birth, I was overjoyed to have Amelia, it was such a special time for us and while I was intervention free (yeah!). And my obstetrician was pretty hands off, which we really enjoyed. It was also reassuring for us to have her around, just in case. We were happy with our choice," **Scarlet Lee, Melbourne, Australia**

ARE BIRTH CENTRES SAFE?

The largest Australian study to date, recently published, looks at the safety of birth centres. Four years of births in Australia (*over 1 million women*) were examined, of which 21,800 women gave birth in a birth center. Women were then matched by risk. This means all women giving birth in birth centres and delivery wards, classified as low risk (*20-34 years of age, no medical complications during pregnancy*), were compared. The rate of mortality to the mother and baby was significantly lower in the birth center women (*both for first time mothers and women having subsequent babies*).[19]

 Mother's Thoughts

"I switched to a birth centre, and it was later in my pregnancy as I was on the waiting list for months. It was just wonderful when a spot became available. You walk into this cosy place where all the midwives wear normal clothes and you make cups of tea and toast and there is really nothing around to remind you of a big scary hospital. They had big baths where I spent most of my labor. I can truly say I loved having Sam. I guess I should have a horror story because everyone else seems to, but I just don't. I gave birth my way and it has made me a stronger person today. Choose your birth options wisely. You choose who comes to your 21st birthday party and wedding because you know that adds to the whole experience. You spend months planning it until it's perfect. You take lots of pictures to remember it and you tell stories about it for years to come. Why should your birth be any different?" **Fredericka Gomez, Queensland, Australia**

ARE HOME BIRTH'S SAFE?

Women who choose birth at home are less likely to need drugs to speed up their birthing time or reduce birthing pain; they are less likely to have an instrumental or surgical delivery, and less likely to tear. Their babies on average are in better shape when they are born and are more likely to breastfeed.

Trials also show that on every other measure, women and their babies are safer at home. The authors of a **2012 Cochrane review** – the medical profession's gold standard analysis - pointed out that planned hospital births are more likely to end in complications, which they blamed on "impatience and easy access to many medical procedures at hospital."[20]

In addition, observational studies suggest that for low risk women, home birth is mostly safer than a hospital birth. A 2011 study of 64,000 UK women, which included serious injuries as well as deaths, found that home birth was marginally more risky for first time mothers (0.93%). Although for a women who'd had children before, she and her baby were as safe at home as a hospital setting (0.53%).[21]

---

[19] Tracy SK, Dahlen H, Caplice S, Laws P, Yueping Alex Wang, Tracy MB, Sullivan E. Birth Centres in Australia: A National Population-Based Study of Perinatal Mortality Associated with Giving Birth in a Birth Centre. Birth 2007;34(3):194-201

[20] The Cochrane Review, Planned hospital birth versus planned home birth 12 SEP 2012, Ole Olsen, Jette A Clausen

[21] P Brocklehurst, Perinatal and maternal outcomes by planned place of birth for healthy women with low risk pregnancies: the Birthplace in England national prospective cohort study *BMJ2011;343:d7400 Published 25 November 2011,*

"The Royal College of Midwives (RCM) and the Royal College of Obstetricians and Gynaecologists (RCOG) support home birth for women with uncomplicated pregnancies. There is no reason why home birth should not be offered to women at low risk of complications and it may confer considerable benefits for them and their families. There is ample evidence showing that labouring at home increases a woman's likelihood of a birth that is both satisfying and safe, with implications for her health and that of her baby."[1]

Some perspectives on mortality rate

Now all this morbid talk is not particularly pleasant or helpful when we are focused on a remarkable and transformational birth experience. Yet, it is often at the **very heart of our fears** and sinks deep within our soul when we make choices on birth. **A fear release on the health and safety of you and your baby is vital to a confident birthing experience.**

Let's put some perspective on the birth mortality numbers. Australia, like many of the prosperous countries prides it selves on providing safe birthing practices for mother and baby, and as such the infant birth mortality rate in 2011 is 0.004%[22] and the maternal mortality rate is 0.007%[23]. To put this in context, the majority of these deaths are due to previously known severe risks and complications *often known prior to the birth*. It is extremely rare for anything serious to happen to a baby or the mother at birth in our modern society.

These figures are similar to **transportation mortality figures** in the same 2011 period. When we take into account approximately the population of same ages as birthing women, the mortality rate in Australia for road mortalities is close to 0.014%[24]. **Therefore, it is slightly more risky to cross the road or travel in a car than give birth.** Yet we do it every day without a second thought and usually without fear. Is it possible that we are putting too much emotion, fear, and even irrationality into to the safety of our birth? Is the perceived 'safety' of your birth affecting your birth choices?

Hypnobirthing understands that birth carries some small risk, just like crossing the road carries a small risk. Yet the power of Hypnobirthing gives you the tools and knowledge to learn to **'look both ways and cross the road safely.'** Your birth tools will provide you with all the information and techniques to make great birthing choices and birth in comfort and peace.

Crossing the road or travelling in a car is riskier than giving birth in a modern country, yet we do this without fear or thought. Hypnobirthing gives you to tools and techniques to 'travel' across the road of birth and make informed and educated choices, so you are likely to have your fulfilling natural birth.

---

[22] The World Bank - Level & Trends in Child Mortality. Report 2011. Estimates Developed by the UN Inter-agency Group for Child Mortality Estimation (UNICEF, WHO, World Bank, UN DESA, UNPD).
[23] The World Bank - Trends in Maternal Mortality: 1990-2010. Estimates Developed by WHO, UNICEF, UNFPA and the World Bank.
[24] Road Deaths Australia 2011 Statistical Summary Bureau of Infrastructure, Transport and Regional Economics Department of Infrastructure and Transport. Australian Government.

Questions to ask yourself

Place of birth

- ☐ Is fear or other people's judgments affecting where I want to birth?
- ☐ Do I feel safest birthing at home or hospital environment?
- ☐ Do I want to give birth in a hospital where the latest technology is available for high risk women and babies?
- ☐ Do I prefer a smaller community or private hospital, even though it may require transferring to another hospital if my baby or I need special care?
- ☐ Do I feel more comfortable in an out of hospital birthing center that is close to a hospital if a transfer is necessary?
- ☐ Do I want to deliver my baby in a hospital setting that has a home environment?
- ☐ Do I prefer to give birth at home in my own familiar comfortable surroundings?
- ☐ How much do I wish to pay for the place of birth?

Care provider

- ☐ Is fear or other people's judgments affecting who I choose as a care provider?
- ☐ Am I 'high risk' and require the skills of an obstetrician?
- ☐ How much money do I wish to pay?
- ☐ Do I feel safer with an obstetrician, just in case I need it?
- ☐ Do I want the support, encouragement and familiarity of a midwife at my birth?

Quick Exercise: Forgetting everything you know, putting aside all questions and concerns, take a deep breath, close your eyes, and visualize the most perfect birth for you.

What does it look like?
How do you feel?
Where are you?
Who is your care provider?

.....*now see what step you can do today to make that a reality.*

PREPARE YOUR BIRTH PARTNER

Choosing the right birth partner

For thousands of years, women gave birth in their own surroundings, with one to one care from loving, experienced women. Traditional midwives were simply women in the community who knew and understood birth and provided women with love, care, support, and advice during their pregnancy.

As you know, in the last 100 years, the culture of giving birth has changed dramatically, mostly moving from home to hospitals. In many circumstances women are no longer given one to one support. Without doubt, this has had a profound impact on the level of confidence and the birth outcome that women experience. Even for those who choose the private obstetrician route, most of the birthing is undertaken by a midwife with the doctor aiming to arrive thirty minutes prior to birth.

Since the 1970s, there has been a shift towards fathers being at the birth. Nowadays it is expected that they are present, regardless of whether they really want to, or in some cases whether they should be there. For many fathers, being present at the birth is a treasured as an awe inspiring event. However, for some, birth can be perceived as an ordeal which they feel obliged to attend, despite the fact that they are unsure of how they can help their partner, or, how they will cope.

There will be some fathers, who haven't completed the Hypnobirthing Home Study Course or even started it. Sadly the thought is, *'Whatever she wants to do is fine and she will tell me what to do on the day.'* While we know that fathers who learn and practice the hypnobirthing techniques, provide the best possible birthing support. We also know that no matter what is said, some fathers will not prepare for birth.

For those fathers who are unprepared for birth, they are often scared, embarrassed and feel out of their depth. As a result, they are pumping out adrenalin (*which the mother will pick up upon*) and heavily rely on the medical team to "do something." These types of fathers are often seeking additional medical intervention during the birthing time, before the mother needs it or when it may not actually be necessary.

Due to these factors, more women are seeking to reclaim their birth experience and are once again seeking support from other women who will support them in their hypnobirthing. Such support includes relatives and birth professionals such as doulas and independent midwives. These women can offer consistent one to one care, which has been clinically proven to reduce the level of intervention, shorten the length of labor and enable the woman to have a better birth experience.

Planning ahead for your birth

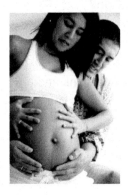

When planning who to have at the birth, it is important that you remember that it is your birth and that you will benefit from feeling as relaxed and confident as possible. You have a choice of who is best to support you on the day.

1. Think carefully about who will give you such support and what support you may want during your birthing day.

2. Have an open and honest discussion with your partner about how you feel. If either of you have any concerns, then discuss alternative options, such as having a close friend, family member or doula to provide additional support.

3. Discuss the kind of things you would and would not like your partner to do.

4. Spend time together preparing for the birth by going through the exercises, listening to the recordings and learning and practicing different techniques and preparing your birth plan.

Birth "support"

Physiologically, a woman needs no "support" to give birth as her body is perfectly designed to birth her baby unassisted. However, she can greatly benefit from **emotional and practical support**, especially when she has chosen to give birth away from familiar surroundings. Key factors to helping her relax and let go would be: feeling safe and unobserved, that her choices are accepted, and that she has focused, continuous care.

Some women benefit from physical support, such as massage or being held, while others may not want to be touched at all. Some mothers gain tremendous encouragement from verbal support, such as being told how well they are doing, or focused counting through each surge, while others will find that distracting.

A woman's needs will also vary according to the different stages of birthing. Often, simply having someone present in the room is enough. However, all women benefit from being free of simple decisions or responding to questions, from minimal distractions and from being in an environment where they feel safe and at ease.

A woman at her birthing time becomes very primal, but also very vulnerable, and so is extremely receptive to the words, feelings and emotions of those around her. She will pick up on the slightest concern, change in mood or body language, even down to the raising of an eyebrow when having her blood pressure taken.

Birth partner as a gatekeeper

As the birthing partner, you may like to view your role as that of her **gatekeeper**. As you know, a birthing woman is essentially a mammal. Think about how animals like to give birth, in quiet, calm environment, warm, relaxed, dim lights, with minimal distractions and intervention.

To have the most natural and comfortable birth as her gatekeeper, your role is to be there:

Physically:

- Attend to her basic needs, such as supplying her drinks, help her to the toilet, bring her a blanket, put a cool cloth on her face, and a hot water bottle for her tummy or back.
- Take care of all practical things, such as taking the bag to the car, calling relatives, bringing enough snacks and drinks for both of you, filling the bath, having change for the car park, petrol in the car and working out the best route to the place of birth.
- Set up the birthing room in the way she would like to be, as homely as possible.
- Some women love to be held or massaged, while others wish to be left alone. Where and how she wants physical support may also change at different points in the birthing.
- Light touch massage to encourage endorphins (see Unit 4).
- Counter pressure massage (see Unit 4).
- Ensure she is being active in her birthing – suggest positions (see Unit 4).
- Other comfort measures in birthing (see Unit 4).

Emotionally:

- Love, support, encouragement.
- Let her know you believe in her strength and power to give birth.
- Remind her of other challenges she has accomplished.
- Trust her to birth in the best possible way for her, even if it is different from what you expect.
- Stay with her, encourage her and express positive beliefs and statements.
- Your attitude and trust in her can make all the difference because her open and vulnerable mind can be strongly influenced.
- Set the pace for relaxation by being relaxed yourself, which is vitally important.
- When speaking to her, recognize that you are communicating with her "birthing mind", which is not in the ordinary everyday consciousness.
- Remember the key to managing her surges/contractions are 'surge breathing' and deep relaxation. Breathe with her if she wishes.
- Use the relaxation trigger 1,2,3,4 relax while putting a hand on her shoulder (practice this often)
- Touch relaxation
- Put on the birth music to encourage relaxation
- If the surges are feeling too powerful and she is in need of more comfort, put on the Anesthesia for Easy Birthing track and encourage her through it (Unit 4).
- If she is nearing transition and in a delicate state of mind and remind her of this time and encourage her gently that she has almost made it, and she will have her baby in her arms very soon.

Among the Peoples of the Yucatan Peninsula, the father is expected to support the birthing mother. This rule is quite stringent, and the absent fathers are blamed for poor birth outcomes.

A great birth partner does not seek to "coach" or tell her what to do, but quietly observes and picks up on her needs and emotions. A great birth partner is present, giving her the encouragement, as well as the physical and mental support, to help her relax and allow her body to birth her baby.

Birth partner's prompts

Some mothers love these and feel really encouraged; others prefer silence and more physical support. At each stage of birthing, the desires of the mother may change. Use these phrases softly in a calm voice.

Between surges – in early and established birthing

- Deepen your relaxation, drift away into relaxation.
- Every muscle is limp and at ease; feel the calm and peace.
- Your body is limp with total relaxation.
- Turn your birthing over to your birthing body.
- Relax and trust your body to know what to do.
- So calm; so comfortable; so at peace.

During surges – softly with direction

- Your body is totally limp; relax into your breathing.
- Trust your body; long, deep breaths.
- Fill the balloon; fill it higher, higher.
- Breathe up, up, up; fill a balloon.
- Your body is limp; arms limp; legs limp, totally limp.
- Fully opening with each new surge sensation.
- Body limp; shoulders limp; chest relaxed.
- Breathe one long breath; work with your baby.
- Baby and mother working effectively together.
- Long, slow breath up.
- Release and relax now.
- Surrender to your body, it knows what to do.
- Your body already knows what to do, just let it be.

During Birth Breathing—lovingly

- Breathe your love down to your baby.
- You and baby working together to bring this miracle.
- Follow the lead of your baby and body, take your time.
- Open the path for your baby.
- Nudge your baby gently down to birthing.
- Your body is following your baby's lead.
- Gently, softly, breathe love down to your baby.
- The path now is open and smooth.
- The baby slips down and out, easily, smoothly.

Mentally: You are the spokesman for her

- Liaise directly with the medical team. Ask the staff to speak to you quietly first outside the room and then if needed, we can discuss the situation together.
- Upon admission, take the responsibility to go through the birth plan line by line with your midwife (*if you are meeting for the first time*) to gain acceptance and confidence that your birth wishes will be respected.
- Ensure medical staff knows to be quiet and not speak to the mother during a surge.
- Medical staff may provide you with lots of information or scenarios that may never happen; it is their way of ensuring you are prepared. Think carefully through any information on how the birthing is progressing.

What if the Medical Team is taking over?

Ask yourself what is more important... having the best possible birth for you and your baby and be good parents, or to be good patients?

Once in the hospital environment, medical teams can be very persuasive, and in some cases even forceful. Remember that they are used to dealing with scared, medicated mothers who have little knowledge of birth and expect to be directed and managed. Nine times out of ten, proposed intervention is not a real emergency and is often more to do with processes, timing, and resources.

What should you do if a midwife or doctor begins putting pressure on you both to "move things along"? Whatever happens, it is vital to stay calm and friendly and never to generate hostility, as a birthing woman simply cannot relax in a hostile environment. The majority of "interventions" are based on protocol or procedures and may not be assessed on a precise evaluation of your individual circumstances.

Laboring scenario

Imagine with me now that a midwife has entered the room and looked at the clock (*again*) and is commenting on the fact that things seem to be going slowly and suggesting that you should perhaps discuss ways to speed things along.

First, stay calm, and ask the following questions:

1. *Is she in any danger?*
2. *Is our baby in any danger?*

If the answers are no, then simply smile, nod, and say,

'In that case, why do we need to rush? Could you please leave us for an hour and we can discuss it again then?'

In the majority of cases, that will be absolutely fine. If there is increased pressure, then it is wise for the birth partners to use questions to help them to make a decision:

Use your 'BRAIN' by asking the following:

B - What are the **Benefits**? - How will this be helpful?

R - What are the **Risks**? - What are the advantages and disadvantages?

A - What are the **Alternatives**? -This may be the routine treatment, but what are different approaches?

I - What does your **Instincts** tell you? - A mother is highly intuitive at birth, trust her choices.

N - What if we do **Nothing**? Why must this be done now? What might happen if we wait another hour or even more?

If you are still not sure, you have the right to ask for a second opinion.

When medical intervention is necessary

Of course, it goes without saying that if there appears to be a strong and conclusive reason for intervention, then that is the time to say thank you to the amazing medical system that we do have. We are extremely blessed to have such wonderful medical support when it is truly necessary, and which ultimately saves lives.

You will know when the medical team need to intervene for your health and your baby's health. Obstetricians and midwives have a **duty of care** to provide you with the best possible treatment and ensure you understand any serious concerns and necessary procedures. If the doctor beliefs that you still do not fully comprehend a serious issue, he or she is duty bound to get another doctor (often a supervisor) in for a second opinion and to help you clarify the situation. As you are under their care and hence their responsibility, they must by law make you fully aware of any serious and life threatening situation, intervention and possible consequences.

Therefore, you are free to ask as many questions as you need, challenge and clarify each situation as it arises. Follow your birth preferences in the confidence that if there is an emergency situation, your medical care givers will always make the situation clear to you, followed by any appropriate action.

Some partners are concerned their written birth choices and questioning the caregivers will stop necessary medical intervention. This is certainly not the case; no matter what the birth plan, medical staff are responsible and held accountable for the health and safely of the mother and baby while in their care.

More comfort measure tools and techniques for birth partners to use are found in Unit 4. In Unit 5 there is a summary of each stage of birthing and how partners can help.

Dad's Thoughts

"This is Michael, Maria's husband. First off, everything is fine. We went in for a thirty-four week follow up ultrasound and the baby was small for that time frame. Turns out "a bit small" meant below where 3% of baby's are at that time. A follow up doctor's appointment to interpret the results led to us going to the hospital for a "day stay" monitoring at 35 weeks. Our appointment was at 11:00 am Thursday morning. After another ultrasound and a flurry of doctor activity, Michael Enrique was born via C-section at 2:20pm on 26th July. He weighed in at 1.8 kilos and measured 42 cm.

Using the B.R.A.I.N. technique really made us feel as we had a "say" and a better understanding of what decisions were being (quickly) made. A C-section was the opposite of how we wanted to deliver, but our little miracle would not have survived being in mom's belly even just another hour and wasn't strong enough for a vaginal birth.

Also, practicing our relaxation breathing techniques turned out to be extremely helpful. It really did calm us while hearing the doctors examine the final ultrasound, while they administered the epidural and during the operation.

Mom is already home and baby will be in the nursery for at least another couple of weeks".

Mike Aquileia, San Francisco, US

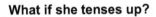

What if she tenses up?

By being so in tune with her, you will also become aware if her manner and disposition seem to change suddenly. This is usually a sign that she is having an **'adrenalin blip',** or is entering the transition stage.

Tensions Signs

- Her breathing changed?
- Her body becomes tense?
- Is she frowning?
- Is her jaw clenched?
- Do her shoulders and neck look rigid?
- Are her toes flexed or curled?
- Are her fingers clenched?
- Are her eyes closed tight?
- Has she becomes more vocal?

These changes can be due to physical stages in the birthing. For example, the surge after her waters release can be significantly more intense. Perhaps it is emotional, such as a fear or concern has appeared.

If this happens, here's what you can do:

- Ask her what has just gone through her mind. Quite often it is a thought which has triggered off the fear and adrenalin. Encourage her to talk about the fears between surges. Do not expect to solve it for her as she may just want you to listen.
- If needed, put on the track 'Release the Fear of Birth' or the 'Quick Release' and let go of the fear.

- If you can remove the source of her fear or disturbance, then do so. She may not like the midwife, or may be disturbed by people coming in and out. You are entitled to ask to change midwives or ask for people to knock and then wait.
- Provide more privacy, ask people to leave the room.
- Avoid unnecessary procedures, such as too many vaginal examinations or over monitoring.
- Change the environment, dim lights, and provide warmth and quiet.
- Use light touch massage to increase the endorphin level (unit 4).
- Use the **relaxation trigger 1,2,3,4 relax** while putting a hand on her shoulder.
- Put on the **birth music** to encourage relaxation.
- Do the '**touch relaxation**' technique.

Mother's Thoughts

"I gave birth three weeks ago.... my waters released on Sunday morning; we ended up staying at home relaxing until 6pm. We got to the hospital and midwives tried to offer pethidine and an epidural however strongly declined with Jim's (husband) support. The pressure got more intense by 2am but then quickly delivered a baby boy at 2.47am with no pain relief. I had no tears and no stitches were needed. After feeding the bub for almost an hour, I was able to jump in the shower with no assistance.

The following days were also amazing as I continually got offers for pain relief but really didn't need it. Midwives were always surprised when I declined pain relief during my stay. I am back at the gym already. **Jasmine Secore, Adelaide, Australia**

UNIT 3: SUMMARY

- **How you breathe** at each stage of your birthing time, will significantly influence your birth for the better or worse. You and your baby deserve the best possible birth experience, so start the preparations now by ensuring each breathing pattern is practiced to perfection.

- **Visualization** gives ourselves a blue print for how we wish things to be, with our body responding accordingly. Harness this power for your amazing birth and visualize each and every stage playing out to perfection.

- **By deepening your relaxation at birth**, you are allowing your body to do its job faster and more effectively. You will find it is easy to surrender to relaxation when you perfect the relaxation triggers and techniques.

- **Where and who you birth** with can fundamentally change the course of your natural birth. Do everything you can now to ensure that your birth choices will be supported.

- **Birth partners are a vital part** of the Hypnobirthing program, without their support it would be a challenge to fulfill your birthing dreams. If your partner is not fully participating in hypnobirthing, then you will need additional hypnobirthing support. You and your baby deserve it!

Skills builder

Quick exercises this week:

- When you first lay in bed at night, spend a few minutes doing relaxation breaths and find yourself drifting off to sleep faster.

- If you feel a stressed moment, consciously stop and take one relaxation breath and feel the difference it makes. The more you do this, the more automatic relaxation will be for you.

- For surge breathing: remember the link between the more you can breathe up into your abdomen, the easier the pressure sensations of surge will be for you? So it is important to practice and continually challenge yourself to breathe as deeply and for as long as you can into your abdomen. Practice five minutes each day.

- After thirty-five weeks, it is useful to practice the birth breathing technique while doing a bowel movement, before thirty-five weeks just focus on learning the birth breathing techniques.

- Set time aside with your partner to practice:

  o   1,2,3,4...relax trigger (with just the phrase and also the hand on shoulder)

  o   Touch relaxation

  o   Hypnobirthing breathing exercises

- With each time you practice, you will find you are more quickly accessing a deeper level of relaxation.

- Soak in a bath with candles and listen to your chosen birth music to deepen a relaxation response every time you hear the music.

Partner's Can Help

- Learn all the tools, techniques, and breathing until they are second nature, then you will best be able to support her on the day.

- Above all else you are her greatest supporter and believe in her power to birth easy and effectively. Demonstrate this to her and encourage her daily.

- Have many of the day to day tasks taken care of, so she can relax effectively of an evening, and eat and sleep well.

- Join with her in the relaxation and breathing exercises, and enjoy seeing a closeness develop between you that will be strengthened at the birth.

- Start communicating effectively with the caregivers and practice the 'B.R.A.I.N' technique now, and see how easy it will then be on the day of the birth.

- All breathing techniques with step by step videos are found on our website at **www.hypnobirthinghub.com/resources**

I know the birth tools: Checklist

☐   Relaxation breathing is easy and I use it anytime I need to find peace and calm

☐   Surge breathing is becoming automatic and 'my balloon' is continually rising up higher

☐   Birth breathing is something I am comfortable with and will practice daily from thirty-five weeks

☐   Perfect pushing (intervention) is practiced in case a 'change of plans' is needed

☐   I have daily set aside time to relax up until my birth – **one** of the following:

  o   Pregnancy health and relaxation track

  o   My own relaxation with Fractional relaxation and progression

  o   Birth music while relaxing in a warm bath or similar

  o   Birth music while performing Relaxation breathing

  o   Partner directed Touch relaxation

☐   My partner and I can perform the 1,2,3,4....Relax trigger

☐   My partner and I are confident with Touch relaxation

☐   I have a special place to use when I am in a surge

☐   I visualize my perfect birth often

☐   I see the 'baby head down' and 'butterfly from cocoon' pictures daily

Unit 3: Hypnobirthing Home Study Course Recordings

 Anesthesia for Easy Birthing

T1 Introduction
T2 Relaxation Triggers and Special Place
T3 Creating Anesthesia for Birthing (Leave for Unit 4)
*Listen **once** to these recordings and you may need to return to these recordings to listen again to create a deeper lasting relaxation trigger.*

 Breathing and Birth Visualization

T1 Introduction
T2 Visualize your Amazing Birth
T3 Birth Affirmations
T4 Relaxation Breathing
T5 Surge Breathing (Contractions)
T6 Birth Breathing

 Audio Guide – Unit 3 (Track 3)

This guide comprises of additional material to support Unit 3 of Hypnobirthing Home Study Course. You can listen once, or as many times as you need. The audio guide is the only recording that you can listen to while you are driving in the car. **Podcast:** *For this free audio track on this unit, go to* http://hypnobirthinghub.podbean.com/ *(Episode 1).*

 Videos: **Hypnobirthing Breathing Techniques**

Step by step guide to easily master the full Hypnobirthing Hub breathing techniques.
These video breathing techniques App can be downloaded for free on both iTunes and Android. Alternatively, these are also freely available on our website.

• Relaxation Breathing, Surge Breathing, Birth Breathing, Perfect Pushing (for intervention)

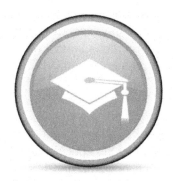

UNIT 4: I HAVE THE KNOWLEDGE FOR BIRTH

The healthy interaction of your hormones and your birth stages are crucial at this time. In this unit, we will examine your body's blueprint for birth and how medical intervention can significantly alter the course of your birth. If circumstances arise and you need an induction, medical pain relief or other intervention, we will examine the best choices to make. We will also look into the many effective and natural alternatives that would work best for you and your baby. In this unit, we also review being active in your birth, and show how this can reduce a birthing time by a third.

The natural stages and phases of birth

It is useful to understand what happens from a physical, hormonal and emotional perspective when a woman gives birth instinctively. As renowned midwife and author Ina May Gaskin says: *"Birth is the Mount Everest of physical functions in a mammal."*

As you are already aware, nature designed birth to be calm and manageable. Having said that, the following is also true for most women:

- giving birth is intense;
- you will feel strong sensations in your uterus; and
- birth is a fluctuation of emotions and bodily changes

However, your state of mind and physical well-being will play an important role in how well you respond to the process. It's a bit like running a marathon: if you go into it unprepared, dreading it, and feeling certain that you will not make it all the way, the chances are that you won't.

By going into the birth feeling positive, physically, and mentally prepared and confident, you are far more likely to manage the sensations and stay in control.

YOUR WONDERFUL BIRTHING HORMONES

When a woman is giving birth, all the activities within her body are dictated by the secretion of hormones. There is an intricate and exquisitely balanced combination of hormones necessary to trigger all functions of labor and birth. When all the birthing hormones are present, the body will go through every detailed stage of birthing with no interference or need for anything outside her body, i.e. medical support or intervention.

It is therefore sad and quite worrying that in modern society, women all over the world are regularly giving birth without the natural secretion of birthing hormones. Instead, birthing women these days are being pumped with chemical, synthesized hormones to "force" the body to go through the birthing process.

It is very important to note that the hormones do more than create the physical functions of birth. Yes, they are responsible for the movement of muscles, the relaxing of ligaments and the expanding of the birth canal, and so on. But the hormones, at the same time, also have an enormous impact on the emotional and mental state of the mother, especially where bonding and love are concerned.

Oxytocin

This is the queen of all hormones. The word oxytocin is derived from the Greek words *okus* and *tokos* meaning quick childbirths. The hormone is nature's way of ensuring the survival of the species, as it is a wonderful incentive to continue to procreate. Oxytocin produces in us such powerful and positive feelings that it has been named as the **"hormone of love"**.

It's the hormone which is released whenever the chemical response of "love" kicks in: during love making, birth, breastfeeding, bonding, cuddling, and so on. The more oxytocin we have in our system, **the more we produce and the better we feel**. The production of oxytocin leads to feelings of calm, wellbeing, patience, lower blood pressure, better digestion and better healing.

Maternal instincts and love

The high levels of estrogen at the end of pregnancy increase the number of oxytocin receptors in the mother's brain in readiness to promote maternal behaviour. This means that by the time your baby is born, your brain has been **"hard wired" for maternal instincts**. During your pre-labor warm ups, oxytocin triggers frequent uterine contractions known as Braxton Hicks contractions.

During your birthing time, oxytocin helps mothers to mentally "go off to a different place" level, allowing the body to take controls. **Oxytocin makes women connect** with the birthing process and feel a **deep love for her baby** as she births.

Oxytocin is the "driver" behind surges

It's the pulsating release of oxytocin which triggers the longitudinal muscles of the uterus to reach down and gently pull open the circular muscles of the cervix. As the uterus contracts, signals are sent to the brain to produce more oxytocin. In turn, it helps the uterus contract more effectively to produce even more oxytocin. This wonderful cycle of triggers and hormone production will continue throughout the birthing time, as long as the mother is not disturbed.

During labor, oxytocin receptors throughout the body are on high alert. These receptors are found in the cervix, birth canal, perineum, vagina, nipples, and even on the skin. Gentle pressure, massage, and stimulation in any of these areas ensure that the production of oxytocin will remain steady and high, **as long as there is no interference from fear-induced adrenalin, drugs or artificial hormones.**

Oxytocin pushes your baby down for you

Once the gap in the cervix is large enough for the baby to pass through, it's fully dilated and the baby's head begins to press down into the birth canal, the receptors there send a new wave of signals. Such signals trigger another surge of oxytocin as the force of the **contractions changes to ones of pushing down (*on their own*)** rather than opening the cervix. Therefore, even in your breathing, your body can actually push your baby down the birth path for you.

The love rush cocktail of birth

At the moment of birth, if a woman is free from chemical manipulation and interference, she will experience a higher level of oxytocin in her body than any other time.

It's perfectly designed to produce an overwhelming feeling of love towards the baby, facilitating the process of "falling in love." There is such a **connection** between a mother and child and it will feel like nothing will ever break that bond. Nature is very clever, as this wonderful feeling is a powerful incentive and driver for a mother to care for her child. Most women report also having stronger connections with their partner's at this time, and a deep feeling of togetherness as a family.

It is also nature's way or rewarding a mother for going through the experience of birth and bringing new life into the world. She will just feel amazing and empowered to do what so many women have done before her. **The feeling is so strong it will stay with her forever**.

> The 'Love Rush' is the best natural 'high' of your life. You will remember and cherish this birth experience for the rest of your life. Nothing will come close.

Oxytocin and the first hour of birth

The vital role of oxytocin doesn't end once the baby is birthed. Once your baby is born, oxytocin continues working as it sends signals to the brain to begin producing milk for the baby. Apart from setting off the message to release the placenta, oxytocin also triggers the uterus to begin to shrink back down again to its pre-pregnancy shape and size.

Skin-to-skin contact with your baby produces even more oxytocin. It's not a coincidence that there is a high concentration of oxytocin receptors in the skin of your chest, meaning that placing your baby on your chest will trigger even more oxytocin. Have you ever wondered why hugging feels so good?

During this time it is vital that the mother and baby are left undisturbed, with as little stimulation as possible. It is also very important to keep the room really warm, as being cold can inhibit the production of oxytocin.

Breastfeeding and Oxytocin

Oxytocin continues to play a vital role in the production of **prolactin** (*hormone for producing milk*) and the bonding process. Yes, we know that the mother also experiences a whole lot of emotional benefits from the hormone, such as having a sense of calm, well-being and patience. With that comes greater production of breast milk, thanks for oxytocin. But it doesn't stop there. Breastfeeding women also benefit from physical changes, including increased functioning of the digestive tract. Being so, they digest food effectively and efficiently in order to produce the right amount of milk for their baby. Equally important, the harmonious relationship between oxytocin and breast milk allows of the increased ability of the mother's body to heal itself.

What destroys Oxytocin

Oxytocin is a very **instinctive and powerful, yet very sensitive** hormone. Any disturbance or interference such as fear, embarrassment, feeling observed or cold can slow down or even stop the production of oxytocin. Medical interventions such as induction, epidurals or anaesthetic injections and the likes, will scare off this wonderful hormone.

Let's face it: there would be times when the release of oxytocin is disturbed. However, the Hypnobirthing Home Study Course provides skills which will enable you to deal with such interruptions or disturbances. Once learned, you can quickly and easily get back on track to an instinctive birth.

Oxytocin, as important as it is, doesn't work in isolation. It's the production of an intricate cocktail of hormones which enables the body to open and release your baby.

Other important hormones include:

Endorphins

Endorphins are the **body's natural painkillers** or opiates. Endorphins are naturally released when the body is involved with physical activity, and especially when there is a level of discomfort or pain. For example, when running or exercising strenuously, the muscles begin to ache and the body produces endorphins. Perhaps when you were having a great time dancing on your new pump shoes or high heels, only to stop and notice some time later that there was a large blister. You didn't feel the pain until you stopped dancing.

Scientists discovered endorphins ("endogenous morphine") in the mid-'70s and found that neurotransmitters in the brain have pain-relieving properties similar to morphine. When endorphins attach to opiate receptor neurons, they reduce the intensity of pain in the human body by naturally blocking pain signals produced by the nervous system.

During the birth, **the flow of the oxytocin triggers the flow of endorphins**. This gradually increases as the labor progresses. By the time the baby is ready to be born, a woman's body is so full of endorphins that many of the sensations are naturally numbed. This hormone actually blocks the pain impulses reaching the brain, thus making the **perception of sensations far less intense**.

Endorphins are also released when a woman is massaged, touched, or deeply relaxed during labor. You will be pleased to know that the Hypnobirthing Home Study Course has a large number of techniques to encourage the natural flow of endorphins during birth.

Relaxin

This hormone is secreted during pregnancy, again building up to a maximum during the birth. It is a wonderful hormone as it helps to make all the ligaments, muscles and tissues soft, supple and stretchy. It helps to soften and relax the ligaments and muscles in the pelvis and the perineum, allowing the bones to shift to accommodate the baby. Relaxin also helps the uterus to become evenly smooth as it expands to accommodate the baby, and at the same time, it helps to soften the round muscles of the cervix.

During the birth, the more a mother breathes in plenty of oxygen and stays relaxed, the higher the levels of relaxin, which help the **birth canal to soften and widen. It also makes a very stretchy perineum,** thus allowing the baby to easily pass through.

 Mother's Thoughts

"I gave birth a year ago now and each time I think back to the birth, I start to well up and have trouble keeping the tears at bay. I know what you are thinking. "Oh, poor girl, she had one of those bad births!" Actually no, just the opposite! It was fundamentally the best experience of my life. Nothing has come close to the overwhelming feeling of gratitude and joy in having such a mesmerizing birth experience. I heard about the love rush that you get when you have a baby naturally, but I don't think anyone really prepares you for just how transforming that feeling is. Every time I look, really look at my baby Hope and she smiles back at me, I get teary all over again as I am transported back in time to her birth. Oh, what a wonderful feeling! I now really know what it is like to have such a strong connection and lasting bond with my baby. I know I would have still had this wonderful connection for Hope if I had an epidural, but I just know that our bond is so filled with joy and has it's foundations on that truly empowering birth and being 'drugged up' on love hormones." **Cindy Chua, Singapore**

Prostaglandin

This is the hormone that enables the cervix to thin and to become the softness of an earlobe. The body will produce this hormone in the **weeks leading up to the birth**. Semen is a natural carrier of prostaglandin and so making love in the build up to giving birth can help to soften the cervix. Also, evening primrose oil and raspberry leaf also help soften a cervix.

THE NATURAL STAGES OF BIRTH

In the final weeks of pregnancy, your body begins its natural preparation for your birthing time. Among the early signs are effacement and dilation. These important changes occur at the cervix and work together to make it possible for your baby to safely and smoothly come out of your uterus.

What is cervical effacement?

Before a women gets pregnant and during most of her pregnancy, her cervix is long and thick. In the final weeks of pregnancy, as the lower part of the uterus gets ready for the baby to come out, the cervix starts to get shorter and thinner. This process is called **effacement**, which is sometimes referred to as "ripening" or "thinning out." As the cervix becomes more and more effaced, it gets shorter and shorter and increasingly "pulled up," eventually seeming to become part of the lower uterus. The cervix itself almost seems to disappear.

As the 'guestimate' birth time nears, the baby's head drops down and the mother's uterus begins to tighten, this, combined with effacement and dilation, can cause pressure and cramp-like sensations. Women, especially those experiencing their first pregnancy, might think this means they're going into active labor. But these pre labor warm ups or Braxton Hicks contractions are just early signs that the process has begun. It usually takes **several weeks for the cervix to become fully effaced**. If a woman is having her first baby, her cervix will probably efface before it dilates; in subsequent pregnancies the cervix may dilate first, then efface.

During the final weeks of pregnancy, your care provider will examine the cervix and can report on these changes. Cervical effacement is measured in percentages. No changes means 0% effaced. When the cervix is half its normal thickness, it's 50% effaced. When the cervix is 100% effaced, that means it's completely thinned out, leaving just the opening at the bottom of the uterus for the baby to come out.

Cervix dilation: getting ready for baby

As the cervix effaces and thins out, it also begins to **stretch and open**. This is called dilation. This widening and opening makes it easier for the baby's head and body to pass through from the uterus into the vaginal canal for delivery.

The degree of dilation is measured in centimetres. For most of your pregnancy, the cervix will be at zero centimetres, closed and not at all dilated, keeping the baby safe and growing inside. The progression of labor is measured by the advancing dilation of the mother's cervix. However, this cannot be generalized for every woman or every pregnancy and can lead to unnecessary intervention.

What triggers your birthing time?

It is thought that when the baby is ready, a message is sent to the brain to start the cocktail of hormones needed for birth.

Labor begins when the **hormone oxytocin** is released. This hormone triggers the muscles of the uterus to begin to flex and tighten, known as a contraction (*surge*). The uterus is the largest bag of muscles in your body and is made up of circular muscles at the bottom, known as the cervix, and longitudinal muscles running down from the top. The longitudinal muscles are soft and supple and reach down to draw back the circular muscles at the bottom gently, just like slowly pulling a polo-neck jumper over your head. If all the other muscles around the uterus are soft and relaxed, then there is no resistance or strain and the opening of the round circular muscles can be done freely and comfortably.

How your cervix gets ready for birth

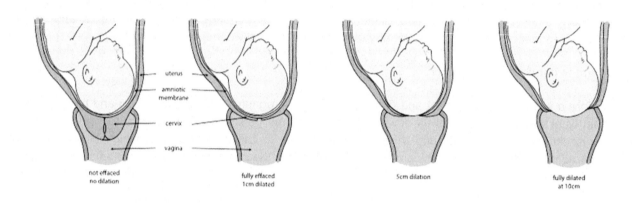

Courtesy Wikipedia, User: Fred the Cybster

How To Know If You Are In Your Birthing Time

You will know when you are - **just trust your instincts**!

Usually, the pattern and frequency of Braxton Hicks changes from infrequent to steady, and it would then seem to follow a **regular and more rhythmical pattern**. The uterus becomes hard during a surge, especially at the top, and you can visibly see when you are having a surge through your stomach and back muscles. If you are in your established birthing then lying down or going for a walk will not stop the contractions, which often happens with Braxton Hicks.

Some women are awakened in the middle of the night with strong regular sensations and just know her birthing time has begun. Others, particularly if pre-labor warm ups have been over days or weeks, it may take longer to realise your body is actually started the birthing time. Your body will tell you when it is happening and give you all the time you need to contact your birthing partner, and slowly and calmly plan your move to your birthing place.

The usual signs of your birthing time

Because every woman is uniquely different, there is a wide range of variations in labor patterns. Early birthing time surges are usually defined as sensations that come every three to six minutes (*timed from the beginning of one surge to the beginning of the next surge*). The contractions (*surges*) are regular, last forty to seventy seconds, and form a pattern that decreases. For example, if contractions are of fifty seconds duration and are six minutes apart. This pattern may continue for nearly one hour and then they become sixty seconds duration and five minutes apart.

As a very rough guide, if you are having surges five minutes apart, it often means you are about four centimetres dilated. At surges two minutes apart, it often means a dilation of seven centimetres.

How to time surges

You will need a watch, or clock, with a second hand and a woman having surges!

- **Time the surges** from the beginning of one to the beginning of the next one, this tells you how far apart the surges are.

- **How long a surge lasts** is from the beginning of the surge until the end of that surge.

- **There is no need to time all the surges** during pre-labor warm ups. This will become tiresome and place pressure on the woman to get into her birthing time. You may wish to time a few surges every few hours to see if a rhythm is developing.

- **Intermittent timing is preferred** over continual timing. Otherwise the main focus will be on the clock (*and for the woman to surge faster*). Continual timing can also distract the partner or support person instead of 'being there' completely for the woman.

- **Your caregiver will usually ask** you how often the surges are coming, and how long they are lasting. The caregiver may stay on the phone while the woman has one or two surges to listen to the sounds she is making and the depth of her breathing. Remember to say you are doing hypnobirthing - so no pain talk!

Unusual signs of labor

Above all, trust your instincts! This is because most women will definitely know they are in their birthing time, yet for some mother's they don't follow the regular pattern of surges. So beware of some of these more unusual signs of birthing.

- **Back sensations** – some mothers only feel the regular surges in their backs and some report the surges as more of a constant dull ache feeling.
- **Strong feelings at the top of the legs**, either continuous or more regular sensations.
- **Braxton Hicks-like surges**, yet very mild sensations which are regular or continuous.
- **Feeling unusual** more focused, emotional and overly connected to your baby (*rush of oxytocin*).
- **Despite any obvious signs** trust your instincts! If you feel it is time, then make your move to your birthing place. If you are wrong, so be it. This mistake happens all the time and it should not be an issue.

When you really need to make a move

There is a general 4-11 rule. Contractions are four minutes apart, last for one minute and for one hour. Yet, everyone is different and often for hypnobirthing women, they are relaxed and plan to go in later. The most important thing is to trust your instincts and if you want to go, make the move when you are ready.

However, here are a few key milestones in the birth journey which your birth partner should look out for and get to your **birthing place sooner rather than later**:

- Your contractions are sixty to ninety seconds and coming every two minutes.
- Your face is continually flushed.
- You have any shaking, vomiting or hiccups.
- You have another bloody show.

- If you feel any rectal pressure or the urge to push, go immediately (*if you live nearby*), or call an ambulance or your midwife and prepare to stay at home.

If you are having a home birth, contact your midwife sooner rather than later. She may come and see you early in your birthing time to provide reassurance, leave for a few hours giving you the privacy you need and then come back when things are more established.

Mother's Thoughts

"With my first baby, I had strong pre-labor warm ups on and off for three days and then on the third day, it was a gradual slide into regular surges. These were just slightly stronger than my Braxton Hicks, but really no different. The second time I knew I was at my birthing time, I woke up at 3am with strong sensations. I knew I was in labor straight away. The surges were 5 minutes apart and lasted for about forty-five seconds. The third time was completely different. I felt like an idiot ringing up the hospital and saying that I wasn't sure if I was in labor. I just had to ring though; there was a trigger inside of me that said 'it's time'. I just felt different and connected to by body and my baby and the sensations I was feeling were really just like regular easy Braxton Hicks.

The midwife said, 'Does it hurt? What's the pain like? Can you talk through a contraction?' I said to the midwife that I did Hypnobirthing with the other two births and they weren't painful, just strong sensations. The midwife said, 'Why don't you call back when you are in pain, dear.' I felt rather patronized, but remembered the Hypnobirthing comment to trust my instincts, so that's what I did. I told Jonathon we are going to the hospital...NOW. He looked a little bemused but complied. When we got there, Jonathon was on strict instructions to stop any questions from the staff on pain and questioning my surges. I needed to stay in my zone and feel positive, believing what I felt was real. On examination, I was 7cm dilated! I felt an enormous sigh of relief to trust my body so completely. And my body didn't let me down now - it was like the baby just slid out. It was the easiest birth ever and the best!" **Larissa Mole, El Pasco, US**

THE BIRTHING TIME PROGRESSION

The progression of labor is traditionally divided into three different stages. The first stage would be when the cervix dilates, the second when the baby is being pushed down and out the birth canal, and the third being the birth of the placenta. In hypnobirthing, we find it more helpful to speak in different terms to make a seamless transition in your birthing time.

In addition to birth stages, there can also be other recognizable phases. These phases usually relate to the intensity of the labor and may become apparent when the woman displays certain emotional and physical signs as her birthing time progresses. Caregivers often look for these signs, to help establish progression of her birthing. **Birth partners also need to be aware** of the changes and responding to different needs during this time.

PRE LABOR WARM UPS

This stage occurs when a woman starts to feel some physical signs that her birthing time could be starting. This could be one sign, or more likely a combination of physical signs, such as a show (*pink or red discharge*), diarrhea (*or loose bowel motions*), nausea, possibly vomiting, backache, period pain, perhaps the waters releasing or some mild to moderate, or regular or irregular surges. During this time, the **cervix softens and ripens, thins out and starts to open slightly** (*or dilate*) up to about one to three centimetres.

Lots of variety in pre labor warm ups

Below are some examples of how pre labor warm ups may emerge before the early birthing time truly begins. These patterns can occur the day you start labor, or two to three days before. It may even be as long as two weeks (off and on) before labor begins.

- Start with **regular surges** that are ten, fifteen, or thirty minutes apart, lasting for approximately twenty to forty seconds. A regular pattern can start to emerge as the surges become stronger, longer and closer together over time, until the early birthing time becomes recognizable.

- Be **strong surges** lasting twenty to thirty seconds coming around five or more minutes apart, or irregular surges perhaps on and off.

- Be a **dull ache** in the lower belly, upper thighs and / or lower back. Some women experience period cramping.

- **Not be particularly noticeable**. You may have slept through most of them during the night, or you may confuse them with the discomforts of late pregnancy.

The emotional side of pre labor warm ups

- The journey to birth can be assessed in several ways. The traditional medical approach uses time and dilation as key measurements. However, every woman is unique and her birthing should not routinely be set against a clock. In fact, it is the use of the **clock in labor** which probably leads to more intervention than any other instrument.

- Using internal examinations is another method used to assess the labor. But then again, the level of dilation has no real bearing on the progress of the birth. Women can be two centimetres dilated for days and not notice that anything is going on. She can go from four centimetres to fully dilated within an hour. **Birth takes as long as it takes**; it isn't to be rushed at all. Your body knows what to do and you will just have to let go and trust it to get on with the job.

- For a first time mother, this initial stage can go on for a very long time. So it is important that you **do not take it too seriously** and get into your birthing mode too soon. If you can sleep, then that is great, or at least go to bed and rest during contractions. If it is "real" labor, it will not stop by lying down. Alternatively, this is actually a good time to do something active such as go for a walk, watch a film, go out for dinner, go shopping or do some baking.

- Some women may find their pre-labor surges difficult to cope with, particularly if they are continuous over a long period. They become disheartened because they are not really in established labor yet. **Focus on the positive** aspects that things are happening; you've waited nine months, and only a little longer.

- Take heart that most of the work is done before the early birthing time. For example, it is not unusual for a woman take two to three days to get to three centimetres dilation in pre-labor, and then only two to six hours for the baby to be born (*once the established birthing starts*). This is why keeping **well-nourished and hydrated** during pre-labor is an important support strategy, so your body can maintain good energy levels to help you birth your baby.

- Pre-labor is exactly that - preparation for labor. The body and the baby beginning, getting ready for the woman to say '**yes' to her birthing time**.

Hypnobirthing and pre labor warm ups

- The best thing at this time is to **get some much needed rest**. The more you sleep and allow your body to do the work for you, the faster this time will pass. Visualize your pre-labor warms up happening at night while you sleep. For many Hypnobirthing mothers, this worked really great!

- **Start your Relaxation breathing** when you need it to provide a sense of calm and comfort. Do a few practice Surge breathing when you feel pre labor warm up surges, to gain some practice for your birthing time, yet too many surge breaths may tire you out over many days.

- It is especially important to **avoid going into hospital/birthing center too soon**, as you are likely to be sent home again (*which is the best thing*). When you stay longer at the hospital or birthing center, you will become open to more intervention as the clock will start ticking as soon as you arrive at the facility. If you are unsure birthing time is really happening, go to the place of your birth. There is no harm in being sent home again for peace of mind.

- **Birth partners**, need to provide all the comfort, attention and understanding in this delicate 'waiting game.' It is a great time to practice comfort measure techniques (*discussed later in the chapter*).

If you have having strong pre-labor warm ups for more than two weeks, check with your caregiver about the position of your baby. If the baby is in a posterior or unusual position, a long pre-labor warm up is the body's way of preparing your muscles and pelvis for a more challenging birth.

EARLY BIRTHING TIME

The early birthing time (*Early Phase 1 in medical terms*) usually occurs when the surges start to become **regular and during this time the cervix is very thin and opens (*or dilates*) to 4 cm**. For some women, this change is obvious. Their surges 'step up,' they become stronger, last longer and are more frequent. For others, it may be more of a subtle change within the woman. Sometimes even the caregiver isn't aware that her labor has taken this change, progressing into a new phase. The change may not be that noticeable because they have been gradual. For many Hypnobirthing women, they don't react very differently to the new sensations of the surges.

Early birthing time surges are:

- **Definite sensations** that start, build up to a peak, and then fade away. The surges become more regular, developing a **definite rhythm**. Surges would be approximately three to five minutes apart, lasting for approximately forty to forty-five seconds.

- The surges could be **mostly strong, long surges** lasting forty to fifty seconds every second or fourth contraction, with mild ones in between.

- Surges that remain **irregular but become stronger**, as you notice the intensity building. These surges may remain irregular (*three to seven minutes apart*) for some time yet.

- Feeling **strong from the very beginning**. Some surges may start with one coming every five minutes (*and lasting forty to fifty seconds*) or you may wake to strong, regular and frequent surges, because you have slept through the beginnings of pre-labor. This is ideal, as you have rested while your body has done some of the work!

- Becoming **stronger after the waters release**, making the surges that follow more intense, more frequent, and longer.

Things to consider in early birthing time

If it is your first baby, usually the early birthing time can take some time. Being so, it's best if you spend this time at home. You may wish to contact your caregiver or hospital delivery suite or birth center staff to let them know that "it has started and is happening." If your partner/s are at work, it may be good to have them at home now to support you as the surges become stronger.

You may also wish to contact any extra support people so they can plan their day (*or night*). For your second and subsequent baby, things can move a little faster, as your body has some memory of 'been there done that!' It is possible to significantly reduce this phase and move quickly to the more transitional phase. In many instances, it still can take some time, so there no need to rush. Take the time you need and calming move to your birthing place when you feel ready to go.

ESTABLISHED BIRTHING TIME (ACTIVE FIRST STAGE)

Now you are fully into your birthing body, usually you will have **past the four centimeters hurdle** as your cervix will now be **quickly opening**, rather than only softening and thinning. At this point you feel like you are really getting on with the business of birthing. By this point, surges are often forty-five to sixty seconds long and three to five minutes apart.

You will begin to feel the need to rest, lie or sit down, or become active between each surge and then move into a comfortable position for the surge itself. These are good, powerful and effective surges. You will now need to concentrate heavily on your surge breathing and use different comfort measures, including relaxation and visualization techniques. You will become totally absorbed and not want to be disturbed. At this point, the more you "let go" and allow your body to get on with what it knows how to do, the better.

Your needs may change rapidly during this stage; one minute you want a massage, the next you cannot bear to be touched. Your birth partner must simply be there for you, accepting how you feel at any given moment.

This is the stage that you will need to make a move to the place of your birth, yet don't make the mistake of going to hospital too soon. This stage can last for many hours, particularly for first time mothers. This is the time to really get primal, and to create a quiet, dark, warm and safe environment, the more you can birth like a mammal, the better.

> Trust your instincts. You usually have an accurate sense of 'when it is time' to call your caregiver, or to leave for the hospital or birth center. As the woman's partner or support, have trust in her instincts. Don't try to move her too early (*to possibly take the pressure / responsibility off you*). Conversely, don't try to keep her at home if she feels too uncomfortable (*or nervous*) about this. She will only labor well if she is feeling at ease, and in control of the decisions.

Established birthing time surges are:

- Your body is working very hard now to open up your cervix. The surges need to be strong to achieve this.
- You will need to focus fully on your surge breathing and relaxation at this stage.
- Your awareness naturally goes inward and become more primal at this time.

- During this time the cervix is opening (*or dilating*) from about four centimetres to around seven to eight centimetres.
- You may need additional comfort measures (*see comfort measures section*).

If established birth surges stop

Travelling or getting ready to move from your home to birth place (*and being anxious or even excited*) can release adrenaline hormones, capable of slowing or stopping surges. For many women, if they are given an hour or so to resettle into their birthing environment and deeply relax, the surges will usually return to their previous pattern. Often setting up the room comfortably, eating or drinking something and waiting calmly a while will see the surges return, as the woman relaxes.

If the surges stop and don't readily restart, you may be presented with the options of:

- Going back home until the surges restart.

- Being able to rest and 'wait and see.' The lull may be a natural resting phase in your labor.

- Being **induced** or **augmented** by releasing the waters or putting up an oxytocin drip. Unless there is a medical reason, be careful of accepting this option, as it will dramatically change the course of your birthing.

> *Induction or augmentation may be the favored choice by some caregivers (especially if they have issues about time limits). Studies have shown that the longer you are in hospital, the more likely the chance that your labor will end up being medically managed.*

Hypnobirthing shortens your birthing time

For non-hypnobirthing women, this established birthing stage often lasts around eight hours for first time and around five hours for women who have had a baby before. The benefit of hypnobirthing and being active at this stage is that it often shortens this stage by two to four hours.

There are two important reasons for this significant time difference;

1. It is proven that **being active during the early and established birthing** time helps prepare a women's body for birth; by helping to position the baby deep within the pelvis and encouraging the pelvis and ligaments to open easily and quickly.

2. With hypnobirthing, a woman welcomes and deeply relaxes with each and every surge; so the surges are much more effective at fully opening the cervix. Therefore **less surges and less time are needed** when compared to non-hypnobirthing women.

Vaginal exams are best avoided

At your place of birth, your caregiver will perform a number of procedures, such as blood pressure, temperature, 20-minute monitoring of your baby, and a vaginal examination to see how far you have progressed. While this initial examination is important, you may like to consider limiting or excluding further vaginal examinations. If you do have internal examinations, it is so important not to focus on the number of centimetres dilated you are.

Many women feel disheartened if they are examined and are pronounced to be four centimetres after hours of surges. It is only our intellectual brain that thinks numbers are significant. What is more important than numbers, is trusting and believing that your body is moving, shifting, softening, tightening and relaxing to get ready for your cervix to open and release your baby.

According to a study published by BioMed Central, the accuracy of vaginal examinations for determining dilation is only 48% to 56% accurate. Moreover, vaginal exams may introduce bacteria into the cervix and can be uncomfortable for some women during her birthing time.

Quick Exercise:

Scenario 1: Let's say you are four centimeters dilated at admission and one hour later, the same midwife comes by and does another vaginal check. She says, 'Great you are five centimeters and progressing nicely. That is what we would expect for you at this time.'

How do you feel? Good! Feels like Hypnobirthing is working. You'd feel calm and confident about birthing.

Scenario 2: The same situation where you are four centimeters dilated at admission and now a different midwife an hour later comes into do a vaginal check. He says 'Oh, still only four centimeters, you haven't moved. We might be in for a long labor! Don't worry, we can always speed things up if things don't change'.

How do you feel? Stressed, anxious and feel a wave of adrenaline pump through your body. Perhaps, feeling that hypnobirthing is not working at all and throw your natural birth out the window!

You are actually the same person in both scenarios with the same vaginal dilation; it is just there is no fully accurate way of assessing dilation. There is no miner's light and a ruler inserted. It is just the pressure the midwife feels on either side of your cervix. This is a very subjective measure and can easily be out by one centimeter from midwife to midwife. By gaining the feedback from your examination, you can unnecessarily change the direction of your wonderful natural birth.

TRANSITION PHASE

The transition phase or end of your established birthing time is often the most mismanaged part of labor. It usually comes in short bursts, often once but sometimes a few times during the later stages of established birthing time (*active stage one*). If you and your birth partner are unaware of this **natural occurring phase**, then it can often lead to unnecessary action being taken such as asking the medical team to "do something" to help.

Having the awareness that this phase is a normal part of your birthing and is in fact an indication that you are progressing really well and close to having your baby can be very reassuring. Once your surges are well established and your body has been gradually opening up for some time, the uterus saves a burst of energy until the last two centimetres for the cervix to open. During this phase, around eight to ten centimetres, the **uterus shifts into a higher gear and surges become more intense** and sometimes feel extremely powerful. **Surges may be sixty to ninety seconds long and two minutes apart**.

It can be a time when you suddenly feel that you are unsure that you will be able to carry on. This usually occurs towards the end of labor and can happen two times. The first can be when you are nearly completing thinning and opening, when your body is moving to the next level, and then again, when your body is almost ready to begin pushing out your baby for you.

The emotional side of transition

You may become more outwardly focused and can experience this sense of whether you can go on much longer. Some women don't actually experience an increase in discomfort during this stage, but they do feel **their emotions have changed**. Your energy is being stored for the final stage and redirected to this area. Many midwives call this transition time of *'the mother's brain in her bottom.'*

Some mothers start to **think a little irrationally** and declare that *"I am going to give birth another day, I have had enough."* Some even start packing their bags and walking towards the door! *"I've changed my mind about having a baby,"* or *"I want to go home,"* and even say, *"Get this baby out of me!"*

Your body may also be showing physical signs that your birthing body is working really hard – hot and cold flushes, shaking, and nausea and vomiting. These are normal physical responses to hard work. Just as when you have run a marathon or carried a heavy object a long way, you can feel hot and shaky or a little nauseous. However, it is useful for you and your birth partner to know about them so that you are not surprised or shocked if they happen.

What to do about it

Mother:

- This is the time to really relax and ride with it. Take each surge for what it is, and focus only on the present moment.
- Remember at all times that you are simply experiencing a feeling, a sensation within your body that you can work with. It can be intense, hard and challenging, but can also be incredible and truly empowering.
- Start to use some of the additional comfort measure. They really do work!
- This phase is only short and will be over very soon and you will be holding your baby in your arms often in fifteen minutes to two hours.
- Remember, some mothers don't have any noticeable transitional period.

Birth Partner:

- Listen attentively to her breathing. You may now have to control the speed of breathing, slow it down, and really concentrate on ensuring her body is really relaxed and limp.
- This is the time to really encourage and praise her. Let her know that she is soon going to give birth to a wonderful baby, that she so close to the end.
- That everything is normal and both she and the baby are OK and doing what nature intended.

Keep the medical intervention at bay

If your birth partner is unaware that this transition phase is normal and to be expected, it is often the **most blundered and badly handled part of birth**. This is because your partner is more likely to seek additional assistance on your behalf. Once you have passed the seven centimetres stage, an epidural usually won't be offered as medical staff knows that in most cases, birthing is nearby and as such there won't be enough time to administer. Usually, with pleading of the partners to *'do something'* an injection of Pethidine or narcotics is given. This only causes an array of problems for the mother and baby.

> *Many women have coped well up until transition, and then suddenly announce they need an epidural. If it is administered, it takes time and many feel the epidural effect only after the baby is born.*

Once you **feel that urge to birth your baby, then all the self-doubt will go** and you will become more energised, determined and so pleased that you passed this stage with flying colours.

Resting time prior to birthing

After transition, there is often a **noticeable break between the surges.** They may even stop for a while. This is a resting phase that can happen as the woman's body re-adjusts to prepare for birthing with the baby getting into the right position for birth. During the resting phase, the cervix is fully dilated (*or pulled completely up into the body of the uterus*). So enjoy nature's way of giving a little respite time before your body births the baby for you.

Releasing of your waters

Your membranes may release their waters (*medically known as 'membranes rupturing'*), at any time during the birth process, even just as the baby is being born. If the waters break at home, check the colour of the amniotic fluid. If it is clear or pink, this is normal. Any green or brownish discoloration could possibly indicate meconium staining. Please contact your caregiver for advice.

The releasing of your membranes occurs mostly (75% of times) when the cervix becomes fully open (*or ten centimetres dilated*), and the baby starts to move down the birth canal. These changes usually put pressure on the bag of waters to burst.

The physical journey of birth

Once the round muscles or the cervix are fully open, the **hormone relaxin** helps the muscles in the birth canal to open. These muscles can spread out and expand to be large enough for a baby to pass through.

Once this happens, the body steps up a gear and the longitudinal muscles begin to push the baby down into the birth canal. **This urge to bear down** or the "foetal ejection reflex" is a natural, instinctive reflex, similar to an overwhelming bowel movement. It's almost impossible to ignore, and to many women it can feel almost pleasurable after the tightening and releasing sensations.

By trusting your body and allowing the urge to bear down to come naturally, your body will do the rest. It is important not to be hurried into pushing, as research has shown that forced pushing brings many negatives to mother and baby.

Once the urge is there, your focus should be on listening to your body, following your 'Birth Breathing' and going with the sensations. Your body will do the rest.

Directed pushing vs birth breathing

Many caregivers will still direct women to push in a certain way. This controlled straining and pushing is known as the 'Valsalva Manoeuvre'. This 'directed pushing' involves being coached to hold your breath for ten or more seconds at a time, and pushing for as long and as hard as you can with only a quick breath in between. This form of pushing can reduce the amount of oxygen available to the baby, increasing the chances of the baby becoming distressed and passing meconium. Women should be encouraged to follow her instincts and birth breath. She only assists her body when it dictates, rather than being coached to push forcefully.

Crowning and birth

Once the baby has moved down through the birth canal, the usually thick layer of concertina-like muscles of the perineum gradually flatten out and cover a much wider area just as the baby is coming out. In addition, the pressure of the baby's head on the perineum reduces circulation which **helps to numb the area**, just like when you sit on your leg for too long and it goes all numb.

Again, nature is incredible, as the cells of the **perineum have more elasticity** than any other part of the body and are flooded with the hormone relaxin to enable them to fan open in order to allow the baby to pass through. At this time, slow down your decent of birthing your baby. It will happen naturally as you allow your baby to rest on your perineum until it is stretched enough for your baby's head to pass through. Remember the butterfly and cocoon visualization picture?

Quick Exercise: *Blow or pant for a few seconds and then add in 'pushing' – similar to doing a bowel movement.*

Did you find it difficult to 'push' and pant at the same time? Most people find it impossible to do both, and that is a good thing. Caregivers will often ask you to blow or pant at crowing, so you can't forcefully push your baby out and tear your perineum.

Remarkably, the baby's head is actually designed to reduce in size as the plates in the skull overlap and the baby's head becomes more oval shaped. As the baby is descending, the pelvic bones also soften and widen (*even more so if you are in a squatting position or upright*).

Cervix in early birthing   Cervix fully dilated

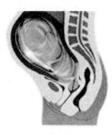
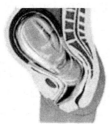

Baby at crowning   Detaching of placenta

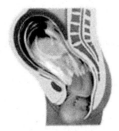
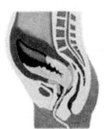

The Stages of Birth

On rare occasions, the waters don't release and the baby may be born with the sac still over their face and head. This is referred to as being born 'in the caul.' Your caregiver will usually break and peel the membrane off the baby's face at birth. Legend has it that these babies have and bring good luck.

The baby's head is usually born with the next surge after crowning happens. With the baby's head now born, the baby instinctively turns its head to allow the easement of the shoulders and body. The woman then waits for another surge before the baby's body is easily born. The baby can then complete the birth journey into the outside world!

Let the cord stop pulsating

After the baby is born, the cord is usually cut to separate the baby from the placenta. The idea being to allow for a resting phase and to clamp and cut the cord after the cord stops pulsating, indicating the placenta has separated. You can feel the cord pulsating in rhythm with your baby's heart rate soon after birth. You may notice your caregiver feeling the cord to make sure the rate is normal.

The cord continues to pulsate until the placenta detaches from the wall of the uterus. The flow of blood in the cord from the placenta to the baby via the umbilical vein continues at a greatly reduced rate for up to five minutes after birth. Minimal oxygen is being supplied at this point to the baby as the baby's lungs take over. By the time the placenta totally separates, the blood in the cord has stopped flowing completely as the cord spasms. The cord is cut at this point or some caregivers cut it after the placenta has been delivered.

The Placenta (Third Stage of Birth)

When the caregiver manages this stage physiologically or naturally, they are flowing with the complex, interconnected process that completes a normal birthing time. Once the baby is born, the natural oxytocin hormone release continues, as the uterus still needs to contract to detach (*and deliver*) the placenta and membranes (*or sac*) that have contained and sustained your baby throughout the pregnancy, labor and birth. The woman's body still has work to do. The surges, although gentler than normal surges, are still needed for the placenta to be expelled to complete the process and to control the bleeding after the birth.

> The more you feel the wonderful rush, love and euphoria in bringing your baby into the world naturally, the more oxytocin you will produce. This means your placenta comes away quickly, safely. In addition, a high level of oxytocin in your system at this time will significantly reduce your risk of excessive bleeding.

It is the first joyous physical contact with a woman's baby that will produce a rush of emotions that are accompanied with a super charged release of her own natural oxytocin hormone. This natural **oxytocin 'surge' or 'rush' makes her uterus contract to cause the separation of the placenta** so it can deliver spontaneously. It is Mother Nature at her finest, including a wonderful oxytocin hormone that floods a mother's emotions with joy, fulfillment, and the deepest form of love and bonding for her baby. Not only does this set up the family unit for life, it has the dual purpose of ensuring your **placenta is detached quickly, easily and safely**.

Once the baby is born, the uterus changes within five to twenty minutes. It immediately begins to contract down, starting the journey of going back to being a small, hollow, pear-shaped organ. As the uterus shrinks down, the small blood vessels which connect the placenta to the mother naturally come away and so the placenta slides away from the edge of the uterus. Once the placenta is no longer attached, the uterus gently expels the placenta, often with one or two easy pushes from the mother.

> *A Lotus birth is leaving the umbilical cord uncut, so that the baby remains attached to the placenta until the cord naturally separates at three to ten days after birth. The long contact with the placenta is seen as a time of transition, with the belief of allowing the baby to slowly and gently let go of the attachment to the mother's body. However this is not a medical preference.*

> (i) *Many traditional peoples hold the placenta in high regard. The Maori people from New Zealand bury the placenta ritually on the ancestral marae. The Hmong, a hill tribe from South East Asia, bury the placenta inside the house of birth and believe the placenta must be collected after death for the next life.*

THE EVERYTHING GUIDE TO INDUCTIONS

On average, one in five women in Australia, UK, and US begin their birth journey by being given chemical hormones which are not their own, prior to the onset of labor. When a woman is induced, the synthetic hormones will produce the desired physical activity, i.e. stimulating contractions in which the uterine muscles flex and release, which in many cases can often be brought on very quickly and with **artificially increased force**. For a woman whose body is not really ready to give birth, induction can also be a long, drawn out process which may take days, making her labor long and tiring. In addition, as this is not a natural process, the **levels of discomfort are artificially higher** than when the body is allowed to gradually build up the strength and rhythm of the surges, supported by natural, comforting hormones.

Induction can be very painful

Many women willingly agree to or even ask for an induction, believing that induction is just like normal labor, just brought on a little earlier. Most women have no real knowledge of the significant differences between natural normal birthing time and one that is induced. One main difference with induction is the synthetic hormones used to start and continue labor. These do not stimulate the body to produce the same levels of complementary hormones, such as endorphins and relaxin and so the **delicate cocktail of hormones is severely disrupted**. As a result, the experience is extremely painful and more difficult for both mother and baby. A labor which is induced is more **likely to need additional intervention**, such as stronger pain relief and subsequently instrumental or surgical delivery.

In spite of this, the number of women being induced has been rising steadily over the last twenty years, even though the World Health Organization recommends that no more than 10% of women should be induced.

What is the induction process?

An induction of labor involves starting a women's birthing time before it starts naturally. It is performed in three ways:

1. Prostaglandin gel applied to the cervix
2. Artificial rupture of the membranes (ARM)
3. Artificial oxytocin (Syntocinon/Pitocin) in an intravenous drip;

One or combinations of these interventions are used to bring on contractions.

Some medical reasons for induction:

- Baby growth restrictions
- Large baby (*be careful how valid this actually is*)
- Placenta dysfunction
- Bleeding in late pregnancy
- Cholestasis of Pregnancy
- Diabetes (*uncontrolled*)
- Epilepsy
- Heart conditions

- Pre-eclampsia
- High blood pressure

It is important to note that inductions can be lifesaving when performed for medical reasons and the benefits outweigh the risks.

Inductions for social reasons

A large number of women are being offered, or even ask for inductions when there is no medical reason to perform one. Quite often their babies are being forced to be born when they are not ready to be born. This, in turn, can lead to a cascade of interventions as it results to additional risks and foetal distress. This is because the body's natural hormones are not able to be released, resulting in the need for further "support".

Some people think that a baby is classed as full-term from thirty seven weeks, and therefore, ready to be born from this period onwards. So then they request to schedule inductions to fit in with home, work or social plans. Be careful in classifying all babies the same as 'full term.' Induced babies prior to forty weeks have a much higher chance of ending up in the special care unit. Some babies are ready to be born naturally at thirty-seven weeks and some well past forty weeks. Just like us adults, **babies are all different from each other.**

There is a growing trend of requesting an induction schedule before forty weeks to fit in with the obstetrician's plans, such as holidays or absences. Perhaps the lure of spending so much money and investing such much energy and trust in an obstetrician can persuade some women to go down this path, often without the full understanding of what they are agreeing to.

 Mother's Thoughts

"When I was thirty-five weeks pregnant with my third child, the obstetrician dropped a bombshell and told me that he was going away on an unexpected holiday over the Christmas period. My baby, Grace, was due on the third of January, and if she came early over the Christmas time, I wouldn't have my obstetrician at the birth. I was so angry and upset about it. He was there for my other two natural and wonderful birth and I was so mad that he might not be there for this one. I felt really betrayed. I know it is a little irrational now, but I am going with the pregnancy brain excuse!

Sensing my distress (not hard, as I had tears running down my face), he suggested an induction before Christmas at thirty-seven weeks. It would guarantee that he would be there for the birth. He said, 'Think about it. You would even be home for Christmas, holding your lovely new baby in your arms. That is a much nicer thought than being in hospital on Christmas day!" I even considered it.

I am so glad that my husband reminded me of why I choose this obstetrician in the first place, as he let me run my own show and have the natural Hypnobirth that I wanted for our first two. Also, my other births were at forty-one weeks, so I had this niggling doubt that Grace wouldn't be ready early. I put on the fear release recording and felt much better about things. I also did a quick release on the need to control my obstetrician. Then, I visualized my obstetrician at the birth at forty-one weeks, having a natural beautiful birth with my husband and best friend beside me.

At 41 weeks and three days, Grace came naturally into the world (birthed by my obstetrician). It was a wonderful, exciting and mesmerising experience. I wouldn't have wanted it any other way. The next day, after the birth, my obstetrician came to visit and said, 'I am so glad that you didn't have the induction, you would have regretted it, I know.' He was right! Hypnobirthing gave me the courage to face my anxiety and have the birth that I really wanted and not selling out". **Donna Switzer, New York, USA**

MANAGEMENT OF PROLONGED PREGNANCIES

In most developed countries, a prolonged pregnancy would be managed by planned delivery through induction. There is **considerable variation in practice between countries, hospitals and obstetricians**. All have different opinions and chosen management styles.

Induction is offered for women who haven't had a previous caesarean. Most women will be offered a repeat caesarean delivery if the pregnancy becomes prolonged, as induction is associated with an increased risk of uterine rupture.

What is a prolonged pregnancy?

Before we go any further let's clarify our definitions;

- *Term*: 'normal' gestation period: thirty-seven to forty-two weeks

- *Post dates*: pregnancy beyond due date: forty weeks plus

- *Post term:* pregnancy has continued beyond term: forty-two plus weeks

Based on World Health Organization [WHO] and International Federation of Gynecology and Obstetrics [FIGO] guidelines, the definition of a post-term or prolonged pregnancy is a gestational age of forty-two weeks or more (*greater than 294 days*) from the first day of the last menstrual period (LMP). As many hospitals have a guideline of induction at forty-one weeks which is before a prolonged pregnancy has occurred, very few women experience a prolonged pregnancy. It is estimated that if induction was not offered, 14% of all pregnancies will proceed beyond forty-two weeks of gestation, while 4% would continue beyond forty-three completed weeks. [25]

Prolonged pregnancy and genetic factors

The idea of a prolonged pregnancy also assumes that we all gestate our babies for the same length of time. However, it seems that genetic differences may influence what is a 'normal' gestation time for a particular woman. Morken, Melve, and Skjaerven (2011) found a familial factor related to recurrence of prolonged pregnancy across generations and both mother and father seem to contribute[26].Therefore, if the women in your family gestate for forty-two weeks, so might you.

Across the world, the median length of pregnancies in **healthy first time mothers is forty-one weeks**. However healthy pregnant women and babies are being offered induction at any time from forty weeks onwards. The irony is that the 'due date' given to women is based on the assumption that all women are the same; that women all have the same twenty-eight day cycle, and that their genetic disposition is the same. However, all women are unique and the duration of their pregnancy will be specific to them. We know that children develop at different rates, so why not accept that some babies may need just that little bit extra time?

Within the developed world the timing and rate of induction varies enormously, with some hospitals routinely inducing at seven days over, some at fourteen days over, and some not having any time related protocol. What does that tell you? This example shows that there is no hard and fast rule about when a woman should, or should not, be induced.

---

[25] Obstetrician/Gynecologist David Barrere, USA 2011

[26] N-H Morken, KK Melve, R Skjaerven Recurrence of Prolonged and Post-term Gestational Age Across Generations: Maternal and Paternal Contribution. BJOG: An International Journal of Obstetrics & Gynaecology Volume 118, Issue 13, pages 1630–1635, December 2011

The point behind this is that, for many women, the medical teams supporting them lead them to believe that these guidelines and procedures are based on non-questionable clinical evidence and in some cases are even compulsory. Many women are feeling like they should be followed without question. **Quite often, the full pros and cons are not given**.

EDD and ultrasounds - have you got your dates right?

Since the 1970s, ultrasound scans have allowed measurement of the size of the developing baby directly and for an estimation of gestation age. Ultrasound dating is most accurate if undertaken in the first trimester (*first twelve weeks of pregnancy*) with a 95% error margin of six days. Scans performed in the second trimester have an error margin of eight days and those in the third trimester a margin of fourteen days.

Most obstetric departments in Australia, Canada, United Kingdom and United States use a combination of LMP (*last menstrual period*) and ultrasound based estimates for the EDD (*estimated delivery date*) using either ten day or seven day rule. This means, that if LMP dates and ultra sonographic dates are in agreement within seven (*or ten*) days, then the LMP dates are accepted.[27] This means there is a **margin of error of up to ten days in calculating estimated due dates**. Therefore, if you are actually thirty-nine weeks and you are incorrectly estimated as forty weeks and three days, you would be offered an induction in many hospitals around the world. No wonder why there are such a large number of induced babies ending up in the special care units.

> Your 'Due Date' could be as much as ten days out. So think very carefully before agreeing to an induction as your baby may not be ready to be born.

The real risk of waiting forty-two weeks or more?

When pregnancy exceeds forty-two weeks gestation, the perinatal mortality rate (*stillbirths plus early newborn deaths*) doubles the rate seen for births at forty weeks gestation[28]. While this increase is statistically small; the actual risk of perinatal death at forty-two plus weeks in Australia and in many other countries is roughly 0.33%. It figures that 99.67 babies out of 100 will be born alive.

Induction carries risk as well; small as it is perinatal death risk of 0.03% (99.97% chance of a live baby). Therefore the absolute risk of waiting and not being induced is 0.3%.

A Cochrane review found that: *"There were fewer baby deaths when a labor induction policy was implemented after 41 completed weeks (42 weeks or later)."* To put this in context, the reports continue to talk about the **option of monitoring post term pregnancies as an alternative policy to induction**"...*such deaths were rare with either policy...the absolute risk is extremely small. Women should be appropriately counseled on both the relative and absolute risks."*

How many women have a discussion with their care provider about the relative and absolute risks of waiting (*with monitoring*) versus induction? Monitoring post term pregnancies is considered a good alternative to induction up until forty-three weeks. The American College of Obstetricians and Gynecologists (ACOG) and many others bodies around the world recommends induction of labor for post-term, low risk pregnancies sometime **during the forty-third week of gestation**.

---

[27] Mittendorf R, Williams MA, Berkey CS, Cotter PF. (1990). "The length of uncomplicated human gestation.". Obstet Gynecol 75 (5): 929–32. PMID 2342739.

[28] Obstetrician/Gynecologist David Barrere discusses post-date pregnancies, 2011

Putting risk in perspective

While these aren't pleasant statistics, we know that it is just **a risk factor and not a certainty** of any kind. Remember back to Unit 3 and the risks about Birth Choices? The same scenario is important to **remove any fear about the timings and choices** that you make when birthing your baby.

There are all kinds of problems associated with providing care based on risk rather than on individual women. However, risk along with due dates are here to stay and women often want to know about risks. Understand that risk is a very personal concept and different women will consider different risks to be significant to them. **Everything we do in life involves risk**. When considering whether to do X or Y, there is no 'risk-free' option. In order to make a decision we need adequate information about the risks involved.

Risks to mothers and babies at 42 weeks plus

One of the most quoted risks to women is the placenta having a limited time span and after exactly forty-two weeks, it starts to shut down. In fact, there is no solid evidence to support the notion that calcification of the placenta is based purely on gestational age.

Some critics also suggest that a baby will grow so big that it will not fit through the birth canal. While some babies will grow significantly bigger (*only 2.5%*), most still will be in the normal range, as it is known that growth generally decreases from thirty-seven weeks. We know that babies, no matter what their size, are pretty good at finding their way out of their mother's expandable pelvis. Think of twins and triplets - they only grow as much as there is space available. In the same way, single babies most of time only grow to fit the designated space available.

> Women are led to believe that induction timings, dates, policies, and procedures are based on worldwide non-questionable clinical evidence. This is not the case! Inductions vary significantly from country, hospital and doctor.

Consider your personal risk:

- **Less effective placenta.** Over time, more calcium is deposited within the placenta, causing it to be less effective. In such case, schedule an ultrasound to detect placenta health.

- **Larger babies.** Only 2.5% exceed 4500grams and thus more risk of mechanical problems in labor leading to Caesarean. How large is your baby?

- **Umbilical cord compression.** This happens if the baby is extremely large and little amniotic fluid. (Schedule an ultrasound to check amniotic fluid levels).

- **Meconium aspiration risk**. If the baby becomes distressed (which is less likely with hypnobirthing.)

- **Poor health, medical ailments and obesity**. These conditions carry more risk.

> *"I have seen signs of placental shut down (ie. calcification) at 37 weeks and I have seen big juicy healthy placentas at 43 weeks."* **Sara Wickham, Midwife and Author**

The brighter future of managing risk

It has been found that many factors other than being over forty-two weeks are associated with an increased risk to the mother and baby. Women with many of these risk factors may be offered earlier induction, but this is not applied in a systematic or consistent way. Conversely, some women have a very low risk despite a prolonged pregnancy and may benefit little from induction[29].

Dr David Bailey suggests we need to **devise customized assessment tools** so that we can estimate the **risk for individual pregnancies**. Women would be offered delivery at a gestation where the estimated risk exceeds an agreed threshold. For an example, an overweight and unhealthy first time woman might be delivered at forty weeks gestation. On the other hand, an uncomplicated woman with a previous birth might be advised against induction at any gestation. This strategy would have the potential to reduce risks without an increase in interventions.[30]

Routine checks reduce inductions

If you are coming close to forty-two weeks gestation and you and your caregiver believe you are low risk, one of the first things you can do is ask for **routine checks to be made on a regular basis**. This is to ensure that you and your baby are both in a good condition.

According to the NICE (National Institute for Health and Care Excellence) guidelines on induction of labor, if you choose not to be induced then you should be offered[31]:

- Twice weekly checks of your baby's heartbeat using an electronic foetal heart rate monitor.
- Single ultrasounds test to check the depth of amniotic fluid surrounding your baby and the health of the placenta.

The aim is to check on the health of your baby, your placenta and your amniotic fluid level. As you reach the end of your pregnancy, your placenta *may* begin to slow down and one of the *first signs* is a reduction in amniotic fluid around the baby. This can correctly be checked by an ultrasound scan. **If those factors are all OK, then there is no reason to be induced**. You can continue to be monitored in this way, every few days until you start your birthing time naturally.

 "It is generally agreed that foetal surveillance in the high risk or post-term pregnancy is associated with a decreased stillborn rate." Dr. David Bailey

Only 5% of births actually occur on their 'due date'.

Please be patient

From the first appointment with your midwife or doctor you will be given a "due date." This date will almost be stamped on your forehead and will be asked of you hundreds of times during your pregnancy. As a result, so much expectation is built up around this date and your mind becomes focused on the birth happening around this time. It can therefore feel like a considerable let down when that date comes and goes.

---

[29] Dr David Bailey, FRANZCOG Management of prolonged pregnancy *O&G* Magazine Vol 12 No 2 Winter 2010

[30] Dr David Bailey, FRANZCOG Management of prolonged pregnancy *O&G* Magazine Vol 12 No 2 Winter 2010
[31] NICE guidelines - induction of labor, July 2008, page 3. Cammu, H. et al.

Other emotions can come into play such as impatience, disappointment and frustration. I have had many mothers to ringing me up one day after their 'due date' in a state of panic. Suddenly they feel that something is wrong with their baby as now are magically past the date. For many women, induction can seem like an "easy" way to have their baby now.

After speaking with your care giver and knowing you are low risk, the **best thing you can do for you and your baby is to wait.** Your baby knows when it is ready to be born and your body will respond as soon as the time is right. Just like an apple falling from a tree, it will only fall when it is truly ripe.

Summary

Induction carries risk and being over forty-two weeks also carries risk. In every part of life there are always risks. But do understand that risks are not a certainty, and it is generally our mind that gives these risks much more credence that they are actually due. Remember all the 'laws of the minds' in Unit 2 and the Fear Releases? If you are scared about going over your 'due date' and think that induction is an easier option. I can fundamentally tell you, it isn't. Induction is like a sentence of 'hard labor' in the Siberian salt mines compared to the 'labor' in tending to your organic nature garden. Don't be tempted to trade in your fear of the unknown for something you may regret later on.

Mother's Thoughts

"Maya was born into water by torchlight. It was a magical moment as she lay on my chest and we stared at each other. I am quietly proud of her birth experience given that I was induced at thirty-nine weeks in a hospital ward.

When I was pregnant, it seemed that just about every birth story I heard ended in an emergency caesarean and I just thought, there is something wrong here. And I researched how to give myself the best chance of a natural birth, and it was at home with an independent midwife. My pregnancy had gone well until about the thirty-seventh week when I became extremely itchy and as it turned that I had Obstetric Cholestasis and needed to be induced early.

Jack and I walked into the hospital on Sunday night. We both wanted to turn and run but we knew it was the best decision for the baby. A lovely midwife booked us in and spent time going through our birth plan and was very understanding that having planned a homebirth, being in hospital to be induced was not where we wanted to be. A young female doctor put the tampon like thing inside me to start the induction overnight. I asked her what was on it and she said "just some medicine". How patronising!!

Firstly, when they broke my waters they said we could go for a little walk – so we went outside and suggested I do some laps of the oval. No seriously!! It was while I was walking that my labor started. I was overjoyed when I felt that first surge - it meant that I didn't need the drip of Pitocin. That was what I so wanted to avoid! Yeah!!

Secondly, Jack asked the head obstetrician, if we could have the monitors on for twenty minutes and off for twenty minutes which he agreed to. This gave me the freedom to move around and I found them extremely uncomfortable on my belly. Thirdly, when they did finally did an internal examination (I held them back as long as I could) I was seven cm. And I heard the midwife say "Yes!!" which gave me a real boost – which would not have been the case if I was only 3cms. Like any endurance activity, the mental aspect is incredibly important.

The hospital had a beautiful big bath and we asked about being able to birth in the water. By then I asked for the lights to be turned off as I really needed to focus inwards and the light was too distracting. I got into the bath and felt instant relief. It was amazing floating in the water between contractions. It was almost like I was sleeping. Before long we realised the baby was coming and they sensitively got a torch so as not to have to put the lights on. She was born without fuss, after only four birth breaths and she didn't cry but just lay on my chest looking at me. It was magic.

P.S. We also felt extremely strongly about letting the cord finish pulsing before cutting it due to the benefits to the baby. The hospital was pushing me to have the Syntocinon injection instead of a 'natural third stage' but Jack talked to the midwife (I was beyond much talking at that point) and he reminded me why we had wanted to do it that way. The hospital was happy to see how it went and I delivered the placenta naturally not long after Maya. It is so important to have someone there to be your advocate and to help you make these decisions so that you can focus on the birth". **Sara Hodgkin, Bristol UK**

NATURAL METHODS OF INDUCTION

There are some things you can do which will not harm you or your baby and may just help to trigger the birth. Some women start these treatments any time after forty weeks. However, you must remember that your baby will only be born when it is ready, and no amount of the following will bring labor on artificially.

Your Birthing Day Guide – This Hypnobirthing Home Study Course recording takes you through each stage of birth and guides your visualizations of this time. The language uses present tense terms such as 'today is the day of your birth' and this guide has helped many women start their birthing naturally. Remember the mind body connection and use it to your advance to bring about the day of your birth.

Acupuncture - The mechanism for acupuncture induction is believed to involve stimulation of the uterus through hormonal changes or direct nerve stimulation, and much research has shown that it can be successful in bringing about contractions[32]. The first records of acupuncture being used for induction of labor come from the Jin Dynasty (AD 265-420)[33]

"Most of the time one treatment is all that is needed to get the process going. Sometimes a second treatment may be needed. Through continual research, we have found that induction using acupuncture generally works within 6-48 hours of having your treatment." **Andrew Orr, Pregnancy and Fertility Acupuncturist, Queensland Australia**

Although acupuncture has been, and still is, a very useful tool for induction, it isn't effective 100% of the time. As they say in China: 'When the fruit is ready, it will fall off the vine.'

Acupressure - Debra Betts has put together a great document on acupressure for pregnancy, labor and post birth, with solutions for all sorts of situations. Details from encouraging labor to reducing vomiting and nausea in labor could be found at **http://acupuncture.rhizome.net.nz/.** If you see a traditional Chinese medicine practitioner, they can show your partner how to apply acupressure as well as treat you at the same time with a variety of great techniques which TCM practitioners use.

Making Love - During love making and especially during orgasm for a woman, the release of oxytocin takes place. In addition, semen contains prostaglandins, a substance which ripens, i.e., softens and stretches the cervix.

Nipple Stimulation - The hormones released when you are physically aroused or during love making are similar to the hormones released during the birth. Therefore, nipple or clitoral stimulation will release oxytocin, which in turn can lead to the uterus beginning to contract, stimulating your nipples (*including your areola, as a baby would when sucking*) with your fingers massaging one at a time. Massage the first nipple for five minutes when there are no contractions, then wait to see what happens (*around fifteen minutes or so*) before doing more.

Evening Primrose Oil (EPO) – This is another 'cervix ripening' method. The oil contains GLA (*gamma-linolenic acid*) which helps the body to make prostaglandins, these soften the cervix and so help the uterus begin to contract. EPO can be used orally and/or internally.

---

[32] http ://www. nice.org.uk/guidance/CG70.
[33] Smith, C. A., 2004, "Acupuncture for the induction of labor ". The Cochrane Data base of Systematic Reviews

A usual oral dosage is two to three of 500mg capsules daily from thirty-six weeks. If you are taking EPO internally, you can do this from thirty-seven weeks before bed time. When doing so, wash your hands well and simply insert two to three capsules as high up into your vagina as you can. You might like to wear a pad or liner as it can get messy when you get up.

Castor Oil – Know that it can cause diarrhea (*and sometimes vomiting*) for the mother which may be unpleasant if you do go into labor. Often in early labor, you will have diarrhea. This is the body's own way of clearing out and making space for baby. But sometimes, this doesn't happen, especially if baby isn't yet ready and given the signal for labor to start. On the other hand, where a post-dates mother had been suffering from terrible constipation and labor had stalled, upon taking the castor oil, she was able to go to the toilet, labor progressed and all went well.

Black Cohosh - This herb is used to encourage contractions and facilitate labor. It should be avoided in pregnancy and is better taken in early labor. Please consult a naturopath before taking as the wrong dose may cause problems.

Raspberry Leaf - A uterine tonic, it also has added benefits after the birth for breast milk production. It's generally recommended any time after twelve weeks in small doses and increased doses from thirty-five weeks. Check with your medical caregiver and a naturopath for doses and to see if it's appropriate for you.

Spicy Food / Curry – Know what it does? Well, spicy food and curry gives some people the runs, so another one to think twice about if this is you! But some women swear by it for getting their labor started.

Induction Massage – This can be given on or after your due date. The massage therapists (who should be experienced in induction massage) work on acupressure points which are normally avoided during pregnancy, which can trigger labor and helps to relax and calm your body, easing tension and helping to create a clear and grounded space. The therapists also may use essential oils which can assist with labor induction.

Eating Date Fruit - A recent study on 'The effect of late pregnancy consumption of date fruit on labor and delivery'[34] concluded that:

> *"The consumption of date fruit in the last 4 weeks before labor significantly reduced the need for induction and augmentation of labor."*

The study included sixty-nine women who consumed six date fruits per day for four weeks prior to their 'due date' and compared the labor and birth outcomes when compared to similar women in gestational age, age and parity, who ate no date fruit. The date fruit group findings were as follows:

- Significantly higher cervical dilatation upon admission.
- Significantly higher proportion of intact membranes.
- Spontaneous labor occurred in 96% of those who consumed dates.
- Use of prostagelatins/oxytocin (for inducing/augmenting labor) was significantly lower.
- Shortens early labor by nearly half.

---

[34] Al-Kuran O, Al-Mehaisen L, Bawadi H, Beitawi S, Amarin Z. The effect of late pregnancy consumption of date fruit on labor and delivery. J Obstet Gynaecol. 2011;31(1):29-31. Jordan University of Science and Technology, Irbid, Jordan

While a larger study size is needed, it is an encouraging outcome.

Walking - The more you can move around, go up and down stairs, walk up hills, the more your pelvis is moving and so the more your baby's head will put pressure on the part of the cervix which can stimulate oxytocin production.

Caulophyllum - Homeopathic Remedy. Only take this remedy once you are at least a week overdue as it is believed to help stimulate surges. It can also be taken during labor for surges which are slow and do not appear to be very productive.

The Cry of a New Born Baby – Visit a friend if you can who has had a new born baby and wait for the cry. The cry is thought to trigger the maternal instincts, which in turn increases the level of oxytocin to start the surges. If you are having trouble finding a new born, watch the movie *Three Men and a Baby*. When the film came out, it made news headlines for bringing on labor.

Globally, in medium-to-large health-care facilities, it is estimated that approximately 10% of all deliveries involve Induction of labor, ranging from 1.4% in Niger to 35.5% in Sri Lanka [1]

INDUCTION: MAKING THE BEST CHOICES

If your caregiver recommends inducing your labor, it is important that you obtain all the facts relating to why the induction is necessary, and exactly how the procedure is carried out. Make sure your caregiver walks you through all the steps **before** being admitted to the hospital, so you know what is involved.

If you feel unsure or uncomfortable about being induced and about the methods being used, then question the reasons around why it might be necessary. Inquire as well if there are any other options available. If you feel you need a second opinion, then follow your instincts.

Stages of Induction

1. Methods to soften the cervix

2. Artificial Rupturing of Membranes (ARM)

3. Artificial Oxytocin Drip – to start contractions

Induction is about **bring your birthing time on earlier** than when your baby would naturally be ready to make their way into the world. Therefore the closer the induction is to this natural birthing time, the more effective and less invasive the induction will be.

In general, many women who have an induction at forty-two weeks, may only need stage one. Others who are at thirty-nine weeks often need all three stages of induction to make it successful. The first two stages can have their own complications, yet on the whole they are a significantly better choice than stage three; the artificial oxytocin drip.

If you have the choice, make the induction as late as possible until your body is close to your natural birthing time. In this way, you have a good change of avoiding the Artificial Oxytocin Drip and have a significantly better birthing experience.

Which induction method?

As the pregnancy draws to a close, the cervix will usually start to soften, thin, move towards the front of the baby's head and open slightly. This is called 'cervical ripening'. The more 'ripe' the cervix is, the more likely it will be to open when the contractions start and the induction successful.

Bishop's Score and induction

To help the caregiver determine which type of induction method is appropriate, they will usually assess the ripeness of the woman's cervix using a scoring system, called the 'Bishop's Score'. Be aware that the interpretation of how the cervix feels (*and therefore the score that is given*) can vary from caregiver to caregiver.

The 4 categories of the Bishop's scoring system are as follows:

1. The consistency of the cervix.

2. The position of the cervix.

3. The thinning (*or 'effacement'*) of the cervix.

4. How engaged the baby's head is.

An 'unripe' or 'unfavorable' cervix is usually not ready to respond to labor contractions. Therefore, it is less likely to dilate in response to certain induction methods, such as an oxytocin drip and breaking the waters. If the cervix does not dilate, the induction is regarded as unsuccessful, and a Caesarean would be required. To increase the success of inductions, medications (*called prostaglandins*) have been developed, aimed at ripening the cervix before the oxytocin drip is given and the waters are broken.

Second or subsequent mothers need less intervention

Women who have experienced a birth before tend to be much more responsive to a wide range of induction methods and are less likely to have an unsuccessful induction. This also means that they usually need less intervention to actually start the birthing time. For example, a woman having her second or subsequent baby is more likely to start her birthing time after just the releasing of the membranes. This is unlikely to be enough to stimulate labor with a first time mother. However, women having subsequent babies are more likely to experience side effects from induction methods using medications. It is for this reason they are usually given lower doses of the drugs than first time mothers.

Methods to soften the cervix

    a) Sweeping the Membranes

    b) Prostaglandins

    c) Foley's Catheter

Sweeping the Membranes

Sweeping the membranes or 'strip and stretch' is an old method of induction that was first documented in the year 1810. It involves the caregiver separating the membranes or sac (*holding the waters and baby*) from their attachment to the lower segment of the uterus. The aim is for your body to **release prostaglandin hormones**. The increased prostaglandin release can be enough to ripen the cervix and make it thin and soft. This is the only induction method that can be given in the doctor's or midwives office. Sometimes this method is enough on its own, and most likely it is the start of the full hospital induction process.

How is it done?

The woman is asked to lie down and the caregiver will place two fingers into her vagina. One of their fingers is placed inside the opening of the cervix, and up just inside the lower part of the uterus, depending on how closed the cervix is and how easy it is for the caregiver to reach. The cervix usually needs to be soft, and slightly open, enough for the caregiver's finger to be inserted. The caregiver then uses a circular sweeping motion (often 360°), to separate the baby's membranes from the lower segment of the woman's uterus. Care should be taken by the caregiver not to break the waters; however, this may happen accidentally.

If the woman's cervix is closed and hence unable to admit a finger, then some caregivers recommend a cervical massage instead, to release the prostaglandins. This would involve the caregiver using their fingers to 'massage' the cervix during a vaginal examination.

Benefits	Downside
Body's natural prostaglandin	Not going to release enough natural prostaglandin if your baby is not ready
Procedure at clinic (no hospital stay)	Possible risk of infection
If it works, hospital induction may not be needed	May risk rupturing membranes
If all goes well, continue with your natural Hypnobirthing birth as planned	Possible uncomfortable, period like cramping or irregular contractions for hours that won't lead to labor
	Possible light bleeding for 24hrs

HOSPITAL METHODS TO 'RIPEN' YOUR CERVIX

If a women's cervix needs to be thinned and softened for an induction, she will be given one of two types of methods to help this process along. The first, a prostaglandin, is a medication, and the second option is a mechanical method called 'Foley's Catheter'.

Prostaglandins for induction

The prostaglandin gel or pessary is placed behind the woman's cervix in her vagina. This is usually done on the antenatal ward *(the floor in the hospital that cares for pregnant women with complications)*. After the prostaglandins are inserted, the woman stays in bed up to an hour, to enable the absorption.

In addition, the baby's heart rate is usually **monitored** for this time with a **CTG Machine.** Prostaglandins have the potential to over stimulate the woman's uterus, causing it to contract too much. The baby can react to this by becoming distressed due to a reduced oxygen supply, and a Caesarean operation may be needed.

Hospital Admission (Antenatal Ward)	Possible Reaction	Risks Factors
Prostaglandin gel, or pessary, placed behind cervix	Over stimulating of uterus, (causing it to contract too much)	Uterus overstimulation more likely if cervix is 'too' favorable, if membranes have released or second or more birth
Bed stay and baby's heart rate monitored for 1 hour, while absorbed	Less oxygen for baby, leading to distress	
	Allergic reaction	If the baby becomes distressed, a Caesarean may be needed.
Second dose given if needed six to eight hours later	Cramping likely	

The Prostaglandin process

The main risk occurs in the first hour of having the artificial prostaglandin absorbed. After this time, the risk is minimal.

Hypnobirthing and Prostaglandins

If the baby is well and the time period of forty minutes or so has passed for the prostaglandins to be absorbed, you will need to stay in the hospital for six hours or more to get the full benefit of the medication. In many cases you will require two doses of prostaglandins (*six to eight hours apart*) to achieve this.

During this waiting time, you may wish to get up and go for a walk. If this is at night, focus on relaxation tracks such as birth music, or the rainbow relaxation track. Most women will experience some cramping, and they may need to use heat packs or a shower for comfort.

In some cases, the surges start soon after and it is common place to be transferred to the delivery suite or birth center. At this point, **take back the control of your birthing and ask to go home**; you are much more likely to then get the birth that you want if you are home during your early birthing time.

Foley Catheter

Using a Foley's catheter to help induce a labor is an old (*but often successful*) mechanical method that can ripen and dilate the cervix. The tip is placed into the opening of the cervix, and the balloon is gently inflated. This puts even pressure on the inside of the woman's cervix. The pressure is aimed at releasing a woman's own natural prostaglandins that can ripen the cervix and/or dilate the cervix to about three to four centimetres. This can take up to twelve hours to achieve. In some cases the catheter will induce the labor contractions. However, often the membranes will be released by the caregiver at some stage, for the labor to keep progressing until the actual birth.

Many caregivers do not have experience in this technique, so check with your care provider. Another similar method is **Laminaria Tents**. Sterile seaweed is introduced into the opening of the cervix, which absorb moisture and gradually swell, to stretch (or dilate) the cervix.

Women who have had a previous caesarean will not be offered Prostaglandins or Artificial Oxytocin. If an induction is needed, give the Foley's catheter a go first before resorting to another caesarean.

Artificial rupture of membranes (ARM)

An ARM is a mechanical way to stimulate or intensify contractions, by placing a hook to break the bag of waters. As the cushion of fluid has gone, this enables the baby's head to press more firmly against the cervix stimulating it to open, and the baby's head to descend further down the birth canal. Some caregivers like to routinely rupture the membranes at some stage during the labor, regardless of whether the woman is progressing slowly or not. Sometimes this is out of habit, in an effort to facilitate as fast a labor as possible. At other times caregivers are curious to see if the water is **meconium stained**, or they would prefer to put an **internal foetal monitor** on the baby's head.

If all women were left to labor naturally, about 75% of them would have intact membranes until they started to felt the 'urge' to birth their baby.

ARM Key Points

- If ARM doesn't start or intensify the labor, then the next intervention is the **oxytocin drip** (Syntocinon/Pitocin) in the delivery suite.

- An ARM has fewer side effects than oxytocin drip, and does not require continuous monitoring.

- ARM done early in the labor (less than three centimetres) gives an increased Caesarean risk, due to **foetal distress.** The natural cushioning of the amniotic fluid usually protects the cord from becoming excessively compressed during the labor.

- An ARM done between three to nine centimetres dilated can rapidly intensify labor sensations, making coping difficult and increases the requests for medical pain relief.

- If the baby's head is lying in an awkward position, the ARM can 'wedge' the baby's head down into the woman's pelvis, before it has a chance to move into a better position, making process slow and uncomfortable.

- An ARM would not be recommended for women with viral infections such as active herpes or HIV/AIDS.

After the ARM has been completed, there is usually no need for continuous monitoring and most hypnobirthing women choose to go home at this stage. If surges have not started or it is early in the birthing time, the best place is to be at home during this time. Many caregivers will give a deadline of twelve to twenty-four hours for the surges to start.

Did you know that when membranes have released either on their own or by ARM, there is a 90% chance of surges starting in twenty-four hours.

Artificial Oxytocin- Syntocinon or Pitocin

Once the cervix is ready for surges to begin, either through your natural hormones to soften the cervix or through the use of prostaglandins, the next step is to start contractions artificially. In most instances ARM has also been undertaken in an effort to give a women's body the best chance to start contracting without the synthetic contraction drug Syntocinon or Pitocin.

To start contractions, an IV drip with the medication is inserted into the vein in arm. The women lays on the bed mostly for the duration of her labor as the drip needs to go through an electronic infusion pump to administers the correct dose of the oxytocin medication and stays in until after the baby is born. A monitor is strapped to the woman's belly to obtain a continuous readout of her baby's heart rate. A CTG machine often relies on the woman being relatively still to obtain an accurate readout. Monitoring is generally conducted from the time the drip is commenced (or the contractions become regular), until after the baby is born.

 Mother's Thoughts

"I was booked in for an induction on April 19th – fourteen days after my official due date. I was so anti induction, but agreed with my OB that if two weeks had passed and nothing happened, I would reluctantly agree. I did all the natural methods possible; yes even the sex (not on my top best sex list!).

Barry and I arrived at the hospital at 7am. We didn't do the gel as my cervix had already started getting ready, so he broke my waters. By midday there were still no surges to speak of, so my OB said we should start the Oxytocin drip. Whoa, slow down....This was the path that I wanted to avoid. Barry stepped in and used the 'B.R.A.I.N' technique and spoke with the OB about going home to see if things started on their own. The OB said 'if you use the Oxytocin drip, you could be holding your baby in a few hours, wouldn't you want that?' It felt really temping you know, like being on a diet for nine months and then waving a Mars Bar in your face. Barry had more strength of character than me at that point (thanks Barry!) and said we will wait and have the birth that we really want.

We put so much effort into learning the Hypnobirthing techniques; we weren't going to give up now! We slept, did the exercises on the ball, walked, chatted and just enjoyed this time together with Brain and the boys. I just loved the surge breathing, when I would go to my special place; a beach holiday that our family took a year ago and it was so special to 'take' my baby into that place. It was like sort of like her 'catching up' on family time.

At no time, was it too uncomfortable and I kind of enjoyed it! Each surge was powerful and my whole belly rose up and tightened. It was pretty cool to show the boys. At the hospital, I was so calm and chilled that they asked me twice whether I was in labor! We went from 6cm to ready to go in two hours. Then when I got this enormous pressure to do a poo, I knew it was time. Barry popped on the birth music and it chilled everyone out. The OB, let me birth in my own time, while I followed my body, just breathing and pushing just a little. Then in twenty minutes our little princess Annalyse was born, chilled and smiling (well not really smiling, but it seemed like it!).

I am so thankful for Barry's strength and negotiating with the OB for us to go home and start things on our own. I know if I had agreed to the Oxytocin drip, it would have been a cascade of intervention and a million miles away from the perfect birth that we worked so hard to get."
Amanda Jordon, Boston, USA

The effect of artificial Oxytocin on you and your baby

When the labor is induced, the medications can sometimes force the **uterus to contract too much**, not allowing the baby recovery time to obtain enough oxygen. This causes the baby to become distressed. As the **baby can become distressed**, continual monitoring is recommended. The mother can also become upset as she struggles to cope with these intense, prolonged contractions.

They can also limit the woman's movement (*often restricted to the bed*) and increase her need for pain relief. If movement is restricted or an epidural is chosen, the labor's progress may be slower or the woman's body will need more oxytocin medications. Sometimes, too much oxytocin can over stimulate the uterus, making it 'contract too much'. An over stimulated uterus can distress the baby, and if this is so, it is more likely the woman will require a Caesarean, **forceps** or **ventouse** delivery.

Continuous monitoring is not always 100% reliable. It can produce a false positive result, meaning babies are identified as being distressed when they are actually doing fine. This can lead to unnecessary interventions ('just in case'), such as a Caesarean.

The pre labor, and early phases are skipped, taking the woman straight into the active phase (or strong, established labor). This does not allow for her body to release natural **endorphins**, natural Oxytocin and hormone helpers to provide comfort. Many women are unprepared for the sudden discomfort and will panic, allowing fear to set in creating the **fear tension pain cycle** making it considerably worse.

The woman's inability to cope leads to **early epidural**s and these can increase the side effects of this form of pain relief and possibly **inhibit the progress of the woman's labor**. This may mean needing more oxytocin to keep the contractions strong, increasing the chances of the uterus becoming over stimulated or 'contracting too much'. An over stimulated uterus can stress the baby. Additionally, with the woman having slow progress, it can increase the chances of her needing more interventions (such as a Caesarean, **forceps** or **ventouse** delivery).

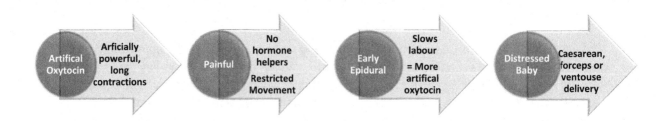

Increased risk of jaundice for your baby

If artificial Oxytocin is used for prolonged periods of time, it makes the baby more susceptible to becoming jaundiced. Large amounts of oxytocin can reduce the amount of salt in the baby's blood, and increase the fragility of the baby's red blood cells. This means that extra red blood cells are broken down after birth. If the jaundice is severe, the baby may need to have phototherapy treatment. Some hospitals perform this treatment in the intensive care nursery, thus separation from their mother is imminent. Other hospitals allow phototherapy on the normal postnatal ward.

You can help by feeding your baby early and frequently. This encourages frequent bowel motions and clears the baby's bowel of **meconium** which helps the baby excrete the bilirubin. By exposing your baby's skin to indirect natural light in the first few days after birth decrease the level of bilirubin.

Premature baby and inductions

As many countries have over a quarter of their babies brought into the world by inductions, it is safe to say that there is a high risk of the baby being premature or not ready to be born. If the induction is done early for medical reasons, then a premature baby may be expected and viewed in these circumstances as an acceptable risk.

We can only guess when babies are due. The best we can do is say that it is sometime between thirty-seven weeks and forty-two weeks. Each individual woman and her baby have their own time clock. This timing may not always agree with the 'official date' given. The earlier the induction, the more likely your baby will be born too early by its own calculations.

Premature babies usually have less body fat and can find it difficult to maintain their body temperature. They may also have a weak sucking reflex and be disinterested in feeding, leading to low blood sugar levels. Treatments can include the baby being cared for in the intensive care unit in an **incubator** to maintain their temperature, and drip in their vein to provide nourishment and increase their blood sugars.

Inductions and clockwatching

Inductions and 'time limits' can often come hand in hand, especially if the waters are broken. Caregivers normally like the labor to be completed within twenty-four hours of the waters releasing, although the actual labor may not start until hours after they are released, even if induced. While the chance of infection may be slightly higher, this is not always the case.

Some caregivers like the convenience of starting an induction at 7 or 8 am, with the baby being born at around 5 or 6 p.m. *(sometimes achievable, but usually an unrealistic expectation)*. This can be one of the 'hazards' of being induced during 'business hours'. Be aware that as silly as this may seem, it is not unknown for a caregiver to walk in at the end of the day, with the statement of "You've had enough time." Then before the woman realizes it, she is being taken to the operating theatre for a caesarean (*or if she is fully dilated*), given a **forceps** delivery to fit in with this schedule. The reason often given in this circumstance is "You haven't progressed fast enough." Some women can be shocked and unprepared for this type of interference. It is important that you discuss such scenarios with your caregiver well before the labor. If you don't agree with their approach, you may choose to change caregivers.

HYPNOBIRTHING AND ARTIFICIAL OXYTOCIN

- To reduce monitoring, request being monitored for twenty minute periods, every hour or two, once the required level of artificial oxytocin is reached (*i.e., your caregiver does not need to increase the dose any higher).

- If you have intermittent monitoring, get off the bed and do all the active birth exercises and comfort measures to help with new strong sensations.

- Once the strong contractions start, hold out for forty-five minutes. This will give your body time to release your some of your own natural **endorphins** and help you cope.

- Remember your Surge Breathing at this time is vital to maintain calm and lessen the strong sensations you feel.

- Perform light touch massage, touch relaxation and importantly the Anesthesia for Birthing. For women who follow these techniques, often find that after this time, they are feeling more relaxed, 'on top of the sensations' and more in control.

Remember, contractions with artificial oxytocin do not feel the same as natural surges. So if you really have trouble coping and have done all you could, it is okay to allow yourself to have an epidural and enjoy the remainder of the birth. It is better for you to have a positive mindset and bond with your baby than to have trauma surrounding the birth.

The emotional side of inductions

If your caregiver recommends an induction, then you may be taken by surprise, raising many emotional reactions.

- Feelings of disappointment in your body and yourself.

- Fear that you are handing over control.

- Upset that you may not be able to give birth where you planned.

- Worried that the induction will be more uncomfortable than you anticipate.

- Unhappy with having to be monitored and restricted in your movement.

- Grief in letting go of how you would have liked the birth to be.

- Feelings of becoming 'a number' in the medical system.

- Feeling concerned or invaded by all the procedures, particularly if you have had past experiences with being touched or examined in a personal or private way by someone you hardly know.

- Worried that you and your baby will be all right, particularly if the induction is happening because of health complications.

Coming to terms with the situation

If the situation doesn't require immediate induction, then you might be able to allow yourself some time to be with your feelings. Talk to your partner or a trusted friend. Identify what is surfacing for you and allow your feelings to be there. Cry if you need to, and explore any alternatives with your caregiver.

Sit with your emotions for the moment, as the worse thing to do is bury the emotions with comments such as "It will be okay", "I'll be alright" "It could have been worse". Yes, you and your baby most likely will be all right, but your feelings should not be negated. Being able to work with your emotions at this time is easier than when they make an unexpected entrance at your birth.

Follow the **Quick Release Technique**, we did in Unit 2 and this will help you find release and acceptance with what is happening. In addition, the following are some things that Hypnobirthing women who needed an induction found helpful.

- **Felt more accepting** of induction if you have tried everything in your power to get into your birthing time on your own which may include some natural therapies or delaying the induction a day or more.

- Remembering that if you have Stretch and Sweep, Prostaglandins, artificial rupturing of membranes or Foley's catheter and **avoid artificial oxytocin**, there is high chance of having a beautiful Hypnobirth.

- **Change your visualization** to that of the natural induction methods working or the less invasive hospital inductions working; surges starting on their own and you going home to continue your hypnobirthing amazing birth.

- **Letting go of the birth you dreamed about**, will help you come to terms with new possibilities and find unexpected joy in your new birthing path.

- **Talking with your partner** and people close to you. Let them know how you are feeling and find out how they are feeling as well.

- **Writing down** (or journalizing) your feelings, fears and disappointments. Then follow the 1,2,3,4 'Release' for each one. You will be surprised how this effective this is.

- **Being aware of all your choices** and being involved in the decisions being made regarding the management of the induction.

- **Sharing your concerns with your caregiver**, exploring other options and gain confirmation about intermittent monitoring and returning home. Look at; **Birthing with Induction – the Birth Plan** to get some ideas on what your preferences are and to discuss these with your caregiver.

INDUCTION SUMMARY

- If you are past due, **double check your dates** in case you may be earlier. This will help many induced (and not ready to be born) babies ending up in special care.

- **Investigate natural alternatives** to induction as much as you can.

- If there are no special circumstances, the **longer you *wait*** *(ideally fourteen days past the due date)*, the more likely your body will respond to induction well. This will maximize your chances of having a baby that is 'due'.

- If your membranes have releases and /or prostaglandins. If they are not successful and surges have not started, go **home again for a few days** before trying again. *(Although many caregivers do not offer this option.)*

- If induction with medications is recommended, you may wish to explore other options to induce your labor, especially if it is your second or subsequent baby. You could consider artificially rupturing the membranes or a **Foley's catheter** before using induction options involving medications.

- If you are prescribed medications, **request for the lowest doses**, and then increasing them slowly. This may take longer but it will reduce your chances of experiencing tonic (over stimulating) contractions.

- Remember to use all the **hypnobirthing techniques** to help you cope with the increased level of sensations. In most cases these are effective to keep mothers free of the epidural.

- **There will be no 'urge' when artificial oxytocin is used**, therefore you will need to rely on vaginal checks to see how dilated you are and rely on your caregivers to tell you when to push. Follow the **'Hypnobirthing Perfect Pushing with Intervention'** method to give you the quickest and most effective method of birthing your baby. This will reduce the need for episiotomy, vacuum or forceps delivery.

- Remember importantly that no matter what happens you are still **in control of your birth and your experiences.** This is equally true for a fully natural birth or an intervention birth. If at any time you are feeling overwhelmed with the change of plans, do the **Quick Release Technique** and feel calmer, confident and in control again.

INTERVENTIONS DURING THE BIRTH

With the increasing medicalisation of birth, many guidelines and procedures are being put in place by hospitals as part of their routine care. Unfortunately, this can often lead to the individuality of each case being overlooked and a blanket approach being used regardless of a particular woman's circumstances. These procedures or guidelines are supposed to be reviewed every five years using the latest evidence based research. However, changes often don't occur. Instead guidelines are still based on the views and practices of individual medical practitioners. In addition, **guidelines widely differ between each hospital, area and even country.**

It is astounding how wide guidelines and procedures differed between countries. For example, in Greenland, epidurals are very unusual at around 8%, while in some hospitals in the US, the rate is over 90%.

"Managed" Third Stage

The birth does not end once your baby leaves your body. The final part of birth is completed when placenta has been released, also known as the third stage.

Now it become commonplace, if not routine in most hospitals, to automatically provide a "managed third stage", i.e., using drugs to speed up the release of the placenta, as opposed to a natural or physiological third stage in which you simply wait for your body to release the placenta. This practice will vary depending where you give birth. Today, birth centres mostly encourage a natural delivery of the placenta, while public hospitals are mixed, and private hospitals under the direction of an obstetrician may routinely manage the third stage.

This "managed third stage" is done by injecting an artificial hormone (pitocin or syntocinon) into a woman as soon as her baby has been born to artificially contract the uterus and release the placenta. The injection is sometimes even before the baby is born as well. Once the placenta is out, the cord is then clamped soon after and gentle pulling of the cord is used to help release the placenta.

The medical benefits of a managed third stage

Once the placenta has been expelled, the caregiver needs to examine it to ensure is has separated cleanly and free of clots. The birth is not over until this stage is done. Therefore, one advantage of medically managing this stage is **the time-saving**. It is about ten minutes for a medically managed third stage, compared to a natural third stage where an average time would be forty minutes. This time-saving would mean less medical time needed at the birth, with resource directed elsewhere.

The drug, the same one used for induction and augmentation, was first used to prevent heavy loss of blood or post-partum hemorrhaging, which can be very serious indeed. In times gone by, this was one of the main reasons women had serious complications after birth, so, when it is truly needed, it saves lives. However, the administration of this drug has now become routine in many hospitals, even when there are no indications that there is potential heavy blood loss or any other medical reason for it. Hospitals tend to be risk adverse, which can be a good thing, yet this often leads to over medical management. In this case, to avoid risks, women are given the artificial oxytocin hormone injection, whether they need it or not.

Why has it become routine?

In the majority of cases, it comes down to training and what the doctor is used to doing. Even though the evidence now says that early cord clamping is not beneficial and possibly harmful to the baby, many caregivers often do what is familiar.

The standard practice for many obstetricians is to cut the cord early for full term babies and allow the cord to stop pulsating for premature babies. The general rationale is that full term babies may not need the blood from the placenta and some think that it may cause some jaundice as the baby breaks down any unneeded blood. However this doesn't take into consideration that the baby will miss out on the many health benefits of the stem cell rich blood.

In addition, caregivers usually are more focused on avoiding additional risks with the placenta, rather than the timing of the clamping of the cord. The standard procedure is to give the artificial hormone injection to the mother as soon as the baby is born. The drug works quickly and could send **powerful surges of extra blood to the baby**. If the baby received an artificially high dose of blood, which would create an **iron overload causing health problems for the baby**. Therefore, if an injection is given and the cord is still pulsating, there will be too much blood for the baby. So, the cord is cut as soon as the baby is born to avoid this iron overload.

Strange as it seems; the artificial hormone injection will give too much blood to the baby, yet **cutting the cord early could reduce the amount of blood in the baby's system by a 1/3.** Wouldn't it be better to wait and see if the mother actually shows signs of medically needing the injection? In this way the baby would be born, the cord allowed to stop pulsating, and receive the correct amount of blood and stem cells. When the cord has stopped pulsating, and then cut the cord. If and only if, the mother needs medical intervention, then the injection can start to work in a few minutes.

> *"Another thing very injurious to the child is the tying and cutting of the navel string too soon which should always be left till the child has not only repeatedly breathed but until all pulsation in the cord ceases. As, otherwise, the child is much weaker than it ought to be, a part of the blood being left in the placenta which ought to have been in the child." Darwin. 1801*

New research and cord clamping guidelines

A Swedish study of 400 children published in the *British Medical Journal* in 2011 found that delaying cord-clamping reduced the risk of a baby having iron-deficiency anemia, which can impair learning development and motor skills.

"The consequences of iron deficiency from early cord-clamping for some vulnerable babies could be serious," says David Hutchon, a fellow of the Royal College of Obstetricians and Gynecologists. *"These range from death, to cerebral palsy, to autism, to Sudden Infant Death Syndrome (SIDS), to slightly lower intellectual ability."*

The National Childbirth Trust agrees, saying the baby's airway should be cleared at the mother's bedside while the baby is still attached by the cord. "We understand that all paediatricians' instincts and training will mean it's hard to wait two to three minutes, but we need to let the cord do its work," says Belinda Phipps, NCT chief executive.

Dr. James Van Hook, director of Maternal Fetal Medicine at the University of Cincinnati Medical Center, says if doctors momentarily delay clamping the umbilical cord, there is a chance that newborns can get a final transfusion of blood cells rich in stem cells and immunoglobulin that theoretically can help the infant fight off infections.

Allergies, immunity and cord clamping

Think back to when you were are child, how many people did you know who had allergies? Most likely it is few. Nowadays, food and environmental allergies are on the increase in many developed worlds.

While the origin of allergies is complex, one factor is thought to be down to the early clamping of the cord at birth. Early studies have shown that babies whose cord has been allowed to stop pulsating before cutting and receive the full stem cells from the cord are more likely to have a stronger immune system and be less likely to develop allergies.

Ever wondered why children in less developed countries have good immune systems and fewer allergies despite poor sanity conditions? In many of these countries they delay the clamping of the cord as standard, thus giving the baby the full quota of blood, oxygen and stem cells.

Interference with your love and bonding hormones

The few moments just after the birth of your baby are when your body produces its highest peak of the love hormone oxytocin and endorphins. This peak in hormone levels is responsible for the natural separation of the placenta from the uterus. It seems the stronger these hormones, the faster, easier and cleanly this separation naturally occurs. In addition to these wonderful hormones, helps you fall in love with your baby and for your body to initiate the breastfeeding process.

If you interfere with this process, i.e. by introducing a synthetic hormone, **your body's own production of oxytocin will be reduced**, which in turn can potentially lead to difficulties bonding and subsequently breastfeeding. There have been studies which have shown that use of syntometrine has led to an increase in difficulties breastfeeding.

It seems that, even when a woman has followed all her instincts and has worked with her body to give birth intuitively and naturally, those precious few moments after the birth of her baby can be interfered due to 'guidelines'.

> *"At the time when Mother Nature prescribes awe and ecstasy, we have injections, examinations, and clamping and pulling on the cord. Instead of body heat and skin-to-skin contact, we have separation and wrapping. Where time should stand still for those eternal moments of first contact, as mother and baby fall deeply in love, we have haste to deliver the placenta and clean up for the next case."[1] Sarah Buckley*

Your third stage options?

The first point is to discuss this with your midwife or doctor and check if you are considered low risk for placenta bleeding. If your risk is no different from other women, explain your wishes to plan for a natural third stage, allowing the cord to stop pulsating then being patient and waiting for your uterus to contract down and release the placenta naturally for you.

You can say that you are happy to adopt a wait and see approach, allowing the cord to stop pulsating and the uterus to begin to contract. However, if there are any signs of heavy blood loss, you are happy to have the syntocinon/pitocin.

Some parents often under the preference of their obstetrician have chosen to wait for the cord to stop pulsating and then elect to have the syntocinon injection once the cord has been cut. In this way, the baby is getting the full benefit of the cord blood and correct blood volume. The additional benefit of this option is that your **natural love rush** has kicked in.

Remember that your body does actually know what to do and given the right conditions, i.e., you are skin to skin with your baby, your baby begins to suckle, you are warm and feel safe and relaxed; the oxytocin will trigger off all the things necessary to release the placenta safely and bring the birth process to its natural end.

Concerns over having a "big baby"

Many women are often told, based on an ultrasound scan, that they are likely to have a "big baby". This can lead to concerns and fears over whether the birth will be more difficult or even possible at all.

The first point to remember is that big babies do not necessarily lead to harder or more difficult births. In some cases, if a baby has a higher birth weight, the birth can actually be quicker and easier, as it is the pressure and weight on the cervix that helps the cervix to open and dilate. Remember that the more gravity and weight there is on the cervix, the more stimulation of the tiny hormone receptors to produce the wonderful oxytocin which makes the contractions even more effective. I have heard so many stories of women who have actually found the births of their heavier babies easier than those of their lighter babies.

Secondly, **ultrasound scans are notoriously wrong** when it comes to measuring the baby's birth weight accurately, often overestimating the weight. For example, one study found that the estimated weight was heavier than the actual birth weight in sixty-six out of eighty-six women studied (77%). A special UK government report concluded that ultrasound estimation of foetal weight was NOT recommended where a large baby was suspected, because the **inaccuracy of ultrasound estimates** has been well documented. Indeed, it is possible that estimating foetal weight by late ultrasound may do more harm than good by increasing intervention rates.

The best advice is that, if you are told you may have a "big baby", you need to assess your own situation, i.e. your size and the size of your baby's father. However, **by nature, your body would not grow a baby that it was not capable of giving birth to.**

You may be urged to have an early induction or a Caesarean section. However, both of these bring additional risks and the evidence does not suggest that they improve the outcome.

One of the main concerns for women having "big babies" is that the head and shoulders may need a little help passing through the pelvis. Simply discuss with your midwives the techniques they use if the baby needs a little help. If people comment on the size of your bump or think you are going to have a big baby, you can simply say, "Yeah, it is great, isn't it? It shows how wonderful my body has been so far in producing such a strong and healthy baby!"

Augmentation

If the clock is ticking and the medical team believe that your labor is taking too long, or your surges have stopped, you will be offered an 'Augmentation.' This simply means stimulating the uterus to contract artificially. Occasionally these drugs can cause the uterus to be what is called 'over stimulated' or contracting too much.

Whether the uterus contracts 'too much' will depend on the woman's individual sensitivity to the drug used and / or whether she has labored before. Women having their second or subsequent labor are much more responsive to these drugs. Overstimulation of the uterus can mean that the baby is not given enough 'recovery time' to obtain adequate oxygen to tolerate the next artificial contraction. This can cause the baby to become distressed and pass meconium. **The drugs for augmentation are the artificial oxytocin drip** and will have the same side effects as the induction drip. (*See Inductions section*)

Remember it is your choice to accept an augmentation or not. Just because your doctor may wear a watch, your baby doesn't. So if you and your baby are OK, take all the time you need to have the birth you truly wish to have. **If your surges have slowed considerably or stopped, ask to go home**. Going home and relaxing in your own environment away from all the pressure to perform, can make all the difference to kick start your birthing time.

Artificially rupturing of membranes (ARM)

Artificially releasing the waters early rather than naturally letting the waters release when they are ready is a mechanical method often used to stimulate surges, especially to induce or augment the labor. Some caregivers like to routinely rupture the membranes, usually during the first stage of labor. This may be done out of habit, or as a way of facilitating a faster labor.

Some caregivers will perform an ARM to confirm if the water is meconium stained. However, routine breaking of the waters can actually **increase the chances of the baby becoming distressed** during the labor. This is because the cushion of amniotic fluid that usually prevents the umbilical cord being compressed unnecessarily during the surges is now removed. Also, the surges are **felt at a greater intensity** as the waters cushion the feeling of the sensations for the mother and her baby. The standard thought is; that if the baby's heart rate is normal, then breaking the waters routinely is not supported for any medical reason.

Waters releasing and infections

In most cases the waters naturally release when the baby is ready to be breathed down for birth. It is unusual for waters to release early without surges, yet it can happen in some instances. What happens next usually depends on the hospital policy and your caregiver's preferences. The guidelines vary considerably from country to hospital to doctor. Some caregivers and hospitals require you to go straight to the hospital. They may also prefer that you be induced within twelve to forty-eight hours if surges don't start. Others administer antibiotics and wait for surges to start. Staying in hospital while waiting for surges to start can put enormous pressure to perform. Being anxious may make it difficult for a mother's body to get into labor naturally. Remember, adrenalin is released when feeling anxious which can suppress surges.

Therefore, many caregivers and hospitals are becoming increasingly flexible with the way they manage pregnant women with released waters. Some allow women to stay at home for twelve to twenty-four hours before coming in for a check-up, particularly if the water is not meconium stained and the baby is felt to be moving. Or come in for a check-up soon after the waters break and then go home again for twenty-four hours or so. A few hospitals opt for daily checks up to seven days before inducing labor, if all seems well. This may happen regardless of whether the waters were slowly leaking or if there was a sudden gush.

If you are well and showing no signs of infection, then there is every reason to wait until your baby is ready to be born, intervention is not needed at this stage. If an infection does occur, it is usually treated effectively with antibiotics, and so removing the need to accept an induction.

About meconium-stained fluid

Meconium stained amniotic fluid is when the baby opens their bowels inside the uterus, making the waters look green, yellow or brownish in colour. It occurs with about 10% of babies who are term (*thirty-seven to forty-two weeks gestation*) and is quite rare if the baby is premature baby (*less than 37 weeks*).

Meconium can be a natural response of a full term baby to opening its bowels. Yet, it also could be the baby's response from a temporarily reduced oxygen supply at some point in time, usually during labor or a slowly reducing level of oxygen over a period of time. Therefore releasing meconium is **one sign** of the baby possibly being unwell or distressed when inside the uterus.

The other sign linked to **lowering/abnormal patterns of the baby's heart rate**. If meconium is seen in the waters, but the heart rate is normal then the baby may not be considered to be distressed. If both are observed, then the perception of distress is more accurate. In addition, meconium can be graded light, moderate or heavy. The majority of meconium stained amniotic fluid is light and is unlikely related to baby distress.

Caesareans

If the baby is showing signs of distress, then the chances of being born by caesarean is increased, if the cervix is not fully dilated. If the mother is in the birthing phase, then the use of **forceps** or a **ventouse** are increased. The decision would normally be based on the baby's heart rate patterns, as well as the thickness of the meconium and when it is first noticed.

A caesarean birth is the delivery of a baby through a cut or incision made by a doctor through the woman's belly and uterus. The placenta is also delivered through the same surgical incision immediately after the baby is born.

A caesarean is a major abdominal operation that can only be performed by a doctor with surgical and / or obstetric qualifications. If a Caesarean is booked before the mother goes into labor then it is termed as an 'Elective Caesarean Section' or a 'Planned Caesarean'. If the caesarean is done after the labor has started it is referred to as an 'Emergency Caesarean Section', even though it may not actually be a true emergency, rather it was unplanned.

Therefore, if someone had an unplanned caesarean, it is always classed as an 'Emergency Caesarean'. Is a true representation of what really went on during the birthing time? If it was a true emergency, then a general anaesthetic is given and the baby delivered quickly, but this situation is rare in hospitals. Most likely it takes one to three hours before the actual caesarean operation is conducted. There will be lots of organisation of staff, the theatre, paperwork, consultations with the Anesthesiologist and forty-five minutes for the medication to work effectively. So, if you hear about an **'emergency caesarean,' in most cases there was never any real emergency. It just means it was an unplanned caesarean.** The difference in terminology can be enormous; one is about fear and the other is just about a change of plans.

Fears of tearing and episiotomy

One of the most common fears for pregnant women is tearing and the need for an episiotomy *(the cutting of the perineum, the skin between the vagina and anus)* during childbirth.

While it is common to have some grazing or superficial tearing, severe tearing or the one that makes us want to cross our legs, is rare. Bad tears, known as third or fourth-degree tears, going all the way from the vagina to the anal opening, are much less common, with a Canadian study finding seven in 100 women suffered a bad tear during birth.

Why an episiotomy might be necessary

There are various reasons why a woman might need an episiotomy, such as her baby is in distress, if her baby is in a breech position and there's a complication, or the birth is progressing quickly and your perineum is at risk of tearing, as it hasn't had time to stretch slowly. The use of forceps does mean that an episiotomy is likely, but not inevitable. A vacuum suction delivery means less chance of an episiotomy, although it may still be necessary. Some doctors say a cut is preferable to the ragged nature of a natural tear. Yet, others say that you never really know if a woman will tear or by how much, just by observation and often episiotomies are done unnecessarily.

Ways to avoid tearing and episiotomies

When your baby's head is about to be born, otherwise known as 'crowning', you'll feel a strong stretching sensation at the rim of your vagina. This is the time that your baby's head is resting on your perineum. The stretching of the skin is white at this time and if you push at this time, you will tear the delicate skin. When the strong stretching sensation lessens, you know you the skin is now pink again and has stretched to accommodate your baby. Pink skin is much less likely to tear.

- Slow down your birth when you feel the strong stretching feeling, wait until this feeling reduces, then gently breathe your baby out.

- Listen to your caregiver. They can see what is going on at this time and will direct you. If there is any doubt, just trust your instincts and wait until you are ready to breathe your baby out at this time.

- Studies show that massaging your perineum, and stretching the skin between your vagina and anus using natural oil, can help prevent tearing when you give birth. Birthing trainers, such as the Epi-no, have the same effect, helping stretch your perineum before birth. (See Unit 1 – Prepare your body in Pregnancy for Birth).

- Water births also help, along with midwives or birth partners pressing warm wet towels on the perineum to reduce tearing.

- Have a bath close to the time of birth; think about your wrinkly stretched skin after your bath, so a long soak in a bath has the same effect.

- Forced pushing, significantly increases tearing. Birth Breathing and being in tune with your body will make a significant difference.

- Epidurals are the number one reason for episiotomies and tearing; as a woman has lost all or many sensations and cannot effectively feel and control the pushing.

- Birthing in an upright or slightly forward position, makes all the difference in keeping your perineum intact.

- Having well developed pelvic floor muscles, as these muscles will naturally hold your baby at crowning, allowing you to wait until your perineum has suitably stretched.

- Add 'no episiotomy' to your birth plan, unless entirely necessary. You have the right to have a local anaesthetic in the perineum before it's done, so insist on that."

Did you know that only 6% of Hypnobirthing Hub mothers having vaginal births had forceps/ventouse/episiotomy or significant tears. That means 92% (the majority) of hypnobirthing mothers who had vaginal births were free from these medical assistance.

Forceps and ventouse

Forceps are like large salad tongs that are wrapped around the baby's head with the obstetrician pulling the baby through and out the vagina. Ventouse (or vacuum), is a similar concept where a cap is place on the baby's head with suction applied to pull the baby out to be born.

These assisted delivery methods are usually used if the baby is already in the birth canal and is thought to be in distress and therefore needs to be delivered soon. They are also used if the baby appears to be 'stuck' in the birth canal. This scenario is common with epidurals and forced pushing, as the mother is often exhausted from all the strain of physically pushing her baby. **It is rare to need forceps or ventouse for a Hypnobirthing woman,** as she follows the lead of her baby and breathes with her body. The birthing muscles work effectively without the need for forced pushing.

If the baby has not started the decent into the vagina, then a caesarean will most likely be needed. If you need an assisted delivery, the choice of how your baby will be born, and the type of method(s) used, will depend on the position of the baby, how far the baby's head has come down the vaginal canal, if you are fully dilated, and the experience and preferences of your caregiver.

In recent years, there has been a swing away from the use of forceps, and a move towards the use of the ventouse. In Europe, the ventouse would be used more frequently than in the United States. In Australia, the use of either will depend on the hospital and the individual caregiver.

Which is the better choice?

- Ventouse is less painful for the mother

- Forceps are painful for the mother and pain relief including an epidural will be offered, if needed.

- While some caregivers will perform an episiotomy for both methods, it is less likely that the woman will tear (or need an episiotomy) with a ventouse.

- It is possible to use a ventouse, if the cervix at least seven centimetres dilated.

- Current research evidence suggests that the ventouse should be chosen first, mainly because it is less likely to injure the woman.

- The ventouse is associated with fewer injuries to the baby's face or head, but an increased chance of developing injuries that clear up in about two weeks.

- Research shows that there are no differences between the ventouse and forceps in terms of the baby's Apgar scores at birth.

- Bleeding in the baby's brain is a very rare complication for both the ventouse and forceps, and can be associated with a difficult delivery, or incorrect application of the devices.

- A headache that lasts one to three days in the baby for both methods.

- An elongated top of the baby's head with a ventouse and indentation marks on the baby's head with forceps. Both will settle in a few days.

Mother's attitude to assisted delivery

While there are risks for the baby with either method, it has been shown that women are more concerned for the health of their baby when a ventouse is used compared to forceps. This is because mothers imagine the effects of the baby being 'sucked out'. This is based purely on the mother's perception of the method used, and not the actual outcome.

Remember that you are unlikely to need any assisted delivery methods when birthing your baby. By giving birth with hypnobirthing, you are using your body to birth your baby for you, by listening and responding accordingly. Forceps, ventouse, episiotomy, and severe tearing are normally a result of forced pushing and intervention.

INTERVENTIONS - MEDICATIONS AND PAIN MANAGEMENT

Although never actually seeing or knowing much about birth, I remember as a teenager having very firm views about medications in birthing. When I was going to have a baby some fifteen years later, I was definitely going to have a caesarean or an epidural at the very least. Why should women be forced into experiencing pain when giving birth, when you don't need to? Isn't birth a medical event, just like surgery? You wouldn't go into surgery for an appendix and say *'I'll like to do this naturally please, no pain relief, thanks.'*

When I was pregnant, thankfully my views all changed. I discovered that birth is not akin to surgery, but rather a natural process of my body to birth my babies. In addition, the most important factor for me was finding out that medications change the delicate hormonal balance and as such, these have a significant effect on the health and safety of myself and my babies.

'Suffer and Serve' was my husband's English grammar school motto. Quite often, well-meaning women say that is just what birth is all about. 'Suffer' extreme pain to 'Serve' your baby. Sadly these women, like martyrs, will deny themselves pain medication to give their baby a better birth experience. These admirable women, unfortunately, haven't heard about hypnobirthing. **There is no need to suffer at all as there shouldn't be any sensation that is too strong to handle.**

With hypnobirthing, it gives you all the tools and techniques so your surges and birthing experiences are comfortable. Therefore it is not that we are asking you to painfully sacrifice yourself for your child - there is just no need to do so. Birth is natural, normal and with balanced hormones and comfort measures, you thrive in your amazing ability of your body to give birth easy, safely and importantly with manageable sensations to give you and your baby the best possible birth experience.

If special circumstances arise in birth and birth now is a medical event, medications can make a significant difference in the emotional and often physical wellbeing of mother and baby. Some medications are a better choice than others, so it is important to have the full information at hand to make the best possible choice. Even though at times in this section, there will be long lists of what could go wrong, remember that for most points **it is just risk, not certainty**. Many women have had these interventions and been free of many side effects. If you need to make a medication choice, focus on being as positive as **you can.**

WHAT ABOUT 'GAS'?

Nitrous oxide, also known as 'laughing gas,' is currently the most commonly used gas for pain relief in labor. It is a colorless, odorless gas that is diluted, usually by half or 50%, with oxygen. In higher levels of up to about 78%, it can be used as part of a general anaesthetic.
Nitrous oxide is absorbed into the woman's blood stream through her lungs and moves rapidly to her brain within ten to fifteen seconds. Once reaching the brain, the nitrous oxide 'depresses' the brain's normal function, **changing how the woman perceives her pain**. It also has a sedative and at times an amnesic effect. The gas is excreted through the woman's lungs as she breathes out. Once she takes the mask away and breathes room air, the nitrous oxide levels rapidly lower with every breath she takes, until none is left in her or her baby's system after a few minutes.

Who shouldn't have 'Gas'?

- Suffered decompression sickness in the past (or 'the bends').

- Had any serious lung problems such as a 'pneumothorax'.

- Feels claustrophobic with a mask on her face.

- Some vegans and/or folate (folic acid) or **vitamin B12 deficiency**. *(The nitrous oxide inactivates these vitamins in the woman's system and in doing so can cause functional disturbances in her spinal cord and nervous system).*

Side effects for the mother

The potential side effects for the woman using nitrous oxide can include:

- **Drowsiness, feeling nauseated or vomiting**

- **Suppression of breathing** – if feeling drowsy, then possible effects on the baby

- **Hallucinations** – including scared or panicked

- Nitrous oxide enhances the effects of narcotic drugs

Side effects for the baby

- Nitrous oxide crosses the placenta to the baby rapidly and the baby has similar side effects to the mother.

- If the baby is noticed to be distressed, the gas may be converted to 100% oxygen for a few minutes and discontinue use. The baby should be OK in five minutes.

- If the mother uses nitrous oxide just prior to birth, it can sometimes affect breathing if the baby is drowsy.

- There is little known about any long term effects on the baby.

Hypnobirthing and 'Gas'

While gas is generally the safest form of medical pain reliever, the benefit is that it will leave yours and the baby's system in a few minutes without long term effect. This means if a mother only used gas for a short time, it is **unlikely to affect the delicate hormone balance** and the mother most likely will still feel the urge to birth their baby.

The downside of gas is that is still a medical intervention and once a women accepts one medical intervention, it is **more likely that she will process to other more invasive interventions**.

 Midwives' Thoughts

"In my 18 years' experience, I have found that the women who do well with the gas are the ones that don't have any particular breathing technique for their contractions. It is so natural and normal to breathe deeply into the belly during a contraction and that is why Hypnobirthing is such a favourite for me. It really provides an inner focus and centre point for the contraction and these Hypnobirthing women do really well with that and keep the sensations under control. The ones who don't know what to do when a contraction comes; pant after the gas, as it forces women to adopt a slow and long breathing pattern. To breathe in the gas, you need to take a deep and powerful breath, like Hypnobirthing Surge Breathing. A few times, I've noticed that the gas canister has run out, but didn't replace it as the women was doing really well with the breathing pattern, but just breathing air!" **Sally Sampson, Glasgow, UK**

WHAT ABOUT NARCOTICS?

A narcotic is a term often given to forms of opiate medications (morphine, pethidine, fentanyl, codeine and heroin). In most countries, including Australia, the narcotic of choice for pain relief in labor is called *Pethidine (known as Meperidine or 'Demerol' in America or 'Pamergan P100' in Europe)*. At times other narcotics will be prescribed, such as morphine, or fentanyl *(known as 'Sublimaze')*.

Narcotics act in a similar way to our body's own natural 'morphine-like' **endorphins**. The medication works by attaching to the nerve fibers in the woman's spinal cord and brain like endorphins, thus reducing her perception of pain. Narcotics are given as an injection into the woman's buttock, leg or arm muscle. **The aim is to reduce *(not eliminate)* strong labor sensations**. A single injection normally lasts three to six hours.

Pethidine tends to be used if the 'gas' has not been effective and the baby is not expected to be born for a few hours yet *(and the woman does not want - or wishes to delay - an epidural)*. Pethidine is discouraged, if labor is progressing rapidly and / or the baby is expected to be born within the following couple hours (although this can sometimes be difficult to predict). This is because the pethidine could suppress the baby's ability to take a breath at birth, especially if given one to five hours before the birth.

Who shouldn't have narcotics

- Not recommended if the baby is premature or suspected of being unwell as side effects cause problems.

- Allergies, intolerances or side effects lasting for several days can occur in some women.

- Pethidine can also interact with some anti-depressant drugs.

- Women who have additions to narcotic drugs in the past may stimulate an addictive response again.

- Women who have built up a tolerance to narcotics will find the standard dose has little effect. Higher doses are not allowed due to possible side effects on the baby.

- Wanting to feel mentally clear and not 'drowsy' or 'drugged'. This effect can vary individually, but the extent will not really be known until the injection is given.

The response of the woman's body in labor and the administration of pethidine is very individual and to an extent very unpredictable. For some women, the pethidine will help their labor to progress; for others it will slow the contractions down.

Side effects for the mother

- **Drowsiness -** Sometimes the mother becomes heavily sedated to the point where she is unable to be easily roused. If she is still affected after the birth, she may be totally disinterested in interacting with or feeding her baby, just wanting to be left alone to sleep.

- **Feeling nauseated or vomiting -** About 15 to 30% of women will find that pethidine makes them feel nauseated and occasionally it will make them vomit. Caregivers may automatically administer an anti-nausea medication mixed with the pethidine.

- **Perspiring** – The narcotic can make the woman perspire or sweat more than usual. Birth partners will need to keep her fluids up, reminding her to drink every few contractions.

- **Suppression of breathing -** Opiates have the tendency to suppress a mother's breathing. In most cases this is mild. If it's a serious concern, for herself and her baby, an injection of **Naloxone** (or Narcan) is given to reverse the effects.

- **Disorientation** – The narcotic can cause confusion, often saying or imagining unusual things. This can make her feel 'out of control', confused and less able to remember the birth.

- **Dizzy** – It can lower the woman's blood pressure and feel dizzy if she gets up quickly. She will need to stay in bed for a few hours after being given pethidine.

- **No natural 'urge'** – There will be absence of the innate urge to birth her baby as her delicate birthing hormones have been medically changed. The mother will then need to be directed to push her baby out.

- **No 'love rush'** – With the narcotic, she will not have the large dose of oxytocin after birthing.

Side effects for the baby

- Pethidine could suppress the baby's ability to breathe at birth, especially if given one to five hours before the birth.

- Usually an injection of **Naloxone** (or Narcan) is given to reverse the effects of pethidine, however the antidote is short lasting and the baby may re-experience breathing problems.

- Baby may require special care or neonatal intensive care from the effects of pethidine, resulting in separation of mother and baby.

- Baby is more likely to have jaundice if their mothers have pethidine.

- Pethidine affects the baby's sucking reflex and can cause breastfeeding difficulties for the first few days.

Hypnobirthing and getting the best from narcotics

Narcotics are certainly not part of a natural birth plan with most Hypnobirthing mothers; they cower at the thought of putting narcotics into their own and importantly their baby's system. However, special circumstances may arise that may make a mother consider this option. If this happens and she chooses to accept narcotics, she needs to remember that:

1. Narcotics affect individuals very differently, including babies. Some people will experience most of the side effects and some will experience one or even none.

2. Take a deep breath and relax then do a Quick Release Technique

3. Think positive thoughts and quickly visualize - you and the baby having the best birth possible with narcotics. Both you and the baby are healthy, happy and doing well.

4. Ask for the lowest does possible (*to lessen side effects*) and increase gradually if needed.

5. If you can, avoid narcotics within a few hours of birth to lessen effects for the baby.

6. Continue with your relaxation and surge breathing. You may find you won't need a top up.

7. Although while you won't have the natural 'urge' to birth your baby, you still can feel the birthing sensations and using the Hypnobirthing 'Perfect Pushing for Intervention' and so significantly lessen the likelihood of a surgical delivery.

EPIDURALS – THE TRUTH YOU NEED TO KNOW

An epidural anaesthetic is an injection of medication(s) administered by an **anesthetist** doctor, into the 'epidural space', usually into the lower (or 'lumbar') area of the spine. Epidurals are a form of what is called 'regional anesthesia'. This means they are aimed at preventing pain sensations (*and to a degree, touch and temperature sensations*) from being felt in the lower 'region' of the body. There are different types of epidurals and often the choice lies with the hospital or individual anesthesiologist.

Three Types of Epidurals:

1. **'Local' anesthetics**, similar to injections used by the dentist, are capable of producing full pain relief for the woman. But this 'local' epidural also have strong side effects and can limit her ability to move in labor or feel and effectively push her baby to be born. These types of epidurals will quickly take effect within fifteen minutes and last only up to two hours.

2. **Narcotic epidural** are found in medications such as Fentanyl, Sufentanil, Morphine and Pethidine (Meperidine in America). These are similar to injections that can be given for pain

relief in labor and after a Caesarean for post-operative pain management. These narcotic epidurals will relieve some but not all labor pain, without causing muscle weakness. This means they usually allow the woman to walk in labor and feel her baby coming down the birth canal to push more effectively. These medications take up to forty-five minutes to have effect and last up to twenty-four hours.

3. **The combined epidural** is the most common type of epidural which is a combination of local and narcotic epidurals. It gives better pain relieving effect, yet increasing the side effects.

Deciding to use an epidural can also lead to a "cascade of intervention," where an otherwise normal birth becomes highly medicalised, and a woman feels that she loses her control and autonomy. Often, the decision to accept an epidural is made without an awareness of these factors and puts significant risks to both mother and baby. Although the drugs used in epidurals are injected around the spinal cord, substantial amounts enter the mother's blood stream, and pass through the placenta into the baby's circulation.

Despite the long list of things that could go wrong with an epidural, it is **just an increased risk and for some women they will experience only a few of these risks on the list**. Therefore, it is not intended to scare, but help you make informed choices.

Side effects for mother (combination epidural)

- Minimal sensations, numb (or 'dead') legs, **inability to stand or walk**.

- **Intravenous (IV) drip** required to counteract a sudden drop in blood pressure.

- Epidural will numb the bladder, and women are often unable to pass urine so a urinary **catheter** is inserted.

- Slowing or prolonging labor; high use of **artificial oxytocin to augment** the labor. This is three times higher in epidurals than non-epidurals.

- Relaxes all muscles including pelvic floor and this can **prevent the baby from rotating** to the correct position in the pelvis, leading to significantly increasing risk of caesarean, forceps or ventouse birth.

- Change the delicate hormone system, so **no 'urge' to birth a baby and directed pushing** is required. This is often very difficult as no sensations are felt.

- 25% of women have very itchy skin.

- 30% of women have vomiting or nausea.

- 33% of women have trouble regulating temperature and shiver.

- Increase risk after five hours of epidural to have a **high temperature and heart rate** for mother and baby, leading to caesarean.

- Choosing an epidural **reduces a standard vaginal delivery** to less than 50% (i.e., without forceps, ventouse or caesarean).

- For ventouse or forceps use, episiotomy is often required. This is where the perineum, or tissues between the vaginal entrance and anus, is cut. Stitches are needed and it may be painful to sit until the episiotomy has healed, in two to four weeks.

The biggest side effect of epidurals

Put aside all the 'maybes' of all the risks just outlined and focus on what I would consider the worst side effect of an epidural. When I welcomed my twins into the world, it was with such an overwhelming joy and excitement with an impenetrable bond with my new born babies. This is the rush of love hormones that gives all unmediated women such a deep lasting and significant satisfaction with the birth process. It is sad to say that women who have an epidural will not receive this **extra 'love rush' and find deep fulfillment in birth**.

Side effects for baby (combination epidural)

- Lowering of the woman's blood pressure which can lead to the baby distress as less blood flow and oxygen are circulating through the placenta. One in eight will be affected.

- A 'non-reactive' **CTG** trace is where the baby's heart rate tends to stay at the same rate *(say around 130 beats per minute)* rather than naturally fluctuating from 120 to 160 beats per minute. This indicated the baby is **'sedated' from the narcotic**.

- Potential to make the baby 'sleepy' and **less likely to want to feed** in the few days following the birth. This is due to their bodies taking longer to eliminate the narcotic medication from their system. At present there are no known long term effects for the baby.

- Risk of rapid breathing in the first few hours and vulnerability to low blood sugar suggest that these drugs have measurable effects on the newborn baby.

- More **difficulties with breastfeeding** which may be a drug effect, or may relate to more subtle changes. Studies suggest that epidurals interfere with the release of oxytocin which, as well as causing the let-down effect in breastfeeding, encourages bonding between a mother and her baby.

- Several studies have found subtle but definite **changes in the behaviour of newborn babies** after epidural with one study showing that behavioural abnormalities persisted for at least six weeks. Other studies have shown that after an epidural, mothers described their babies at one month as more difficult to care for.

Some benefits of epidurals

- If the labor has been prolonged and the woman is exhausted, then an epidural is offered to enable her to rest. The resting may be enough to restart effective surges and avoid augmentation.

- For some women feeling concerned about their birthing time, it can cause anxiety to the point where the fear – tension – pain sets in preventing their birthing from progressing. Often, this rest reduces anxiety and surges can begin again.

- Occasionally, the baby is in a difficult position and despite all natural and Hypnobirthing comfort measures, the sensations are too difficult to manage.

> *If you feel you have done all you can to avoid an epidural and still feel you need it, the worst thing you can do is 'beat yourself up' about it. It is better to greet your baby with joy, love and comfort rather than extreme discomfort and too exhausted even to hold your baby.*

Hypnobirthing and getting the best from epidurals

While we wish and plan to have to have a natural and non-medicated birth, sometimes we have to let go of our ideal birth and accept the special circumstances and make the best of the situation we find ourselves in. Undeniably there are is a long laundry list of things that can go wrong with an epidural. The flip side of that is to **focus on everything that can go right** when having an epidural. Remember your positive thinking and the laws of the mind? If you do come to this situation in the hospital, firstly take a deep breath and then do a Quick Release Technique.

When you are feeling in control and centred once more, have a discussion with your doctor about a **'narcotic or 'walking' epidural**. While this doesn't give superior sensation control, it does help considerably with much less side effects of other epidurals. This type of epidural also has the benefit of less monitoring and the ability to have a more active birth. Although while you won't have the natural 'urge' to birth your baby, you still can feel the birthing sensations and using the Hypnobirthing 'Perfect Pushing for Intervention' and so significantly lessen the likelihood of a surgical delivery.

Importantly, **visualize your best possible birth** with an epidural. This may include feeling calm, relaxed and in comfort. Surges are strong and effective, with no augmentation needed, and perfectly pushing your baby into world on your own. As you bring your baby to your chest, feel deeply loving and connected to your baby as this will **add some oxytocin** to your body, making breastfeeding and bonding easier.

Epidurals and dissatisfaction of birth experience

While an epidural is certainly the most effective form of pain relief available, it is worth considering that ultimate satisfaction with the experience of giving birth may not be related to lack of pain. In fact, a UK survey which asked about satisfaction a year after the birth found that despite having the lowest self-rating for pain in labor *(twenty-nine points out of 100)*, women who had given birth with an epidural were the most likely to be **dissatisfied** with their experience a year later.

Some of this dissatisfaction was linked to long labors and forceps births, both of which may be a consequence of having an epidural. Women who had no medical relief and received their 'love rush hormones' reported the most pain *(seventy points out of 100)* but had high rates of **satisfaction**.

Interestingly, women who do hypnobirthing have the **best of both worlds**, high satisfaction with birth and low pain levels. Wouldn't that option be the best to choose?

ACTIVE BIRTHING IS EASIER BIRTHING

In an 'Active Birth,' the mother herself is in control of her body. She moves and changes position freely as she feels the need to do so. In contrast, in an actively managed birth, all the choices are taken from her and body is controlled and she is a passive patient. An active birth is one where the first resort is the mother's own instinctual and natural resources and the last resort is medical intervention.

When birth is active, you are encouraged to stay out of lying on the bed in your birthing time. Instead of the bed, sit upright on a chair leaning forward, kneeling on all fours on the mat or over the ball, or standing and walking. It's easy to move your body in response to the surges by bending and swaying, circling your hips, or rocking forward and back. Alternatively, you may settle into a comfortable position sitting or kneeling, propped up by lots of pillows, so that your partner or midwife can massage your back, shoulders or feet. When your body is relaxed and free to move, your surge breathing becomes deeper and more effective.

Lying on the back goes against the anatomy of our birth canals. Our human birth canal is actually shaped like a "J" and not a straight line. The baby doesn't just slide straight down and out. It comes down, then up and over the pelvis. Actually, it seems bizarre to think that lying flat on your back with your legs up is an effective way to birth a baby.

In fact, choosing to lie on your back as your main childbirth position **closes your pelvic** area by about 30%. It is no wonder then that those women who follow active birthing positions during the birthing time will **shorten the birth on average by about a third to a half** when compared to women who lay in the bed for their labor and birth.

Simple props such a mat on the floor, a chair, a beanbag, a low stool or a birth ball can help to support you comfortably in these 'gravity effective' positions. You may well find your midwife will be encouraging you to use them and may even provide them for you. This means that you are free to be led by your own powerful intuition, to move spontaneously and guide your baby through the birth canal in the most effective way through your natural movements.

How an active birth works for you

During your birthing time, your baby's head moves slowly down deeper into the pelvic canal as it emerges from the dilating cervix. In these positions, your pelvis is at the best possible angle for gravity to help the process. Numerous studies have shown that this is likely to make labor shorter and more efficient.

Reduces sensations to a comfortable level - The uterus naturally tilts forward. If you are in a more upright position and slightly forward, the uterus has more space than if you were laying down. In this position, the **uterus has more effective surges and the sensations reduce**. Women who are free to move into these positions are less likely to need medical pain relief.

Reduces your baby's distress - There is better blood flow to the placenta when you are upright and breathing deeply. Your baby receives plenty of oxygen this way. There is no compression of the internal blood vessels as there may be if you lie for an extended period on your back or in the semi-reclining position. Foetal distress is a common cause for a caesarean section or the use of forceps or ventouse to deliver the baby quickly. Blood flow to the placenta and the baby is optimal in upright positions.

Birthing is faster and easier - When you are ready to give birth, the kneeling, squatting or upright seated position will help you to use your energy effectively. It is much more powerful to aid your body with the help of gravity and the rotation and descent of the baby's head is easier.

The laying down or reclining position on the bed is, by far, the least beneficial as it works against gravity and reducing the space within the pelvis. When you are upright, the pelvic joints are unconstricted as they would be lying down and this allows a degree of movement and expansion of the pelvis. With this, the internal shape of the pelvis can accommodate the baby's head with maximal space as it descends in labor. At birthing, the back wall of the pelvis (sacrum and coccyx) is free to move back, increasing the diameters of the pelvic outlet to make plenty of space for your baby to come out.

Partners are Involved and Supportive - In an active birth, partners are often more involved in giving both emotional and physical support. This sharing of the birth experience can be very fulfilling and memorable. It is also a good start to a new relationship as parents and the start of your new family. In addition, as the back is more exposed, it is easier to perform massage techniques and other comfort measures.

Reduced Birth Trauma –The baby is born quickly and easily and less likely to suffer trauma during labor and birth. As the baby is likely to be born in optimal condition, bonding after birth and the first breastfeeding are facilitated. Equally important, the mother feels good and recovers well from the birth. This makes caring for the new born baby easier.

> *By staying active and alternating your position from sitting, standing, kneeling and lying on your side during labor, you can decrease the length of your labor (from three to ten centimetres dilation) by up to 50%* [1]

Getting the most out your active birthing time

- Although delivery rooms have beds, remember lying on your back slows down your birthing time.

- To bring additional comfort to a surge, lift your bottom and leaning forward with the surge.

- If you need to rest, rest with your feet **lower** than your bottom to keep your pelvis open. *(i.e. sitting in a chair or a ball is better than sitting in a bed).*

- Warm water can be very soothing and assist mobility. You may be able to be monitored in water.

- Rocking is often comforting and if you need continuous monitoring, then you can still be in the upright position.

- If progress slows your midwife may encourage you to walk upstairs sideways to help your labor along or try kneeling on one knee.

- Your pelvis will open wider if your knees are **lower** than your hips.

- Work with your midwife to find the right support to help you stay upright.

- Change your position regularly as your labor progresses, you may need to ask your birth partner or midwife to help you.

- When you are in your established birthing time, you will probably find that you don't want to move around a great deal, that's fine, you will naturally find the position that suits you best. You may want to be active during your surge, or you simply may want to find the best position to relax and focus on your surge breathing.

> Remember all the exercises that you learnt in Unit 1 and have been doing every week? These are the same active birth exercises that you will use on the day of your birth. If you haven't been doing these exercises, get of the chair and start now!

POSITIONS FOR LABORING OUT OF BED

Walking, Standing and Leaning

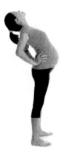

Upright positions for childbirth use gravity to the mother's advantage. They help the baby drop into the pelvis and prevent pressure from being concentrated in a particular spot. They also allow the birth companions to apply other comfort measures easily. Even though you will want to be sitting or off your feet while having a surge; standing, walking and leaning between your surges will help stimulate more effective surges.

Walking is helpful in shortening early birthing, yet you will need to stop and be supported during the surges.

- Stand against a wall for support.
- Have your partner support you as you stand. Let your partner stand behind you and place arms under your arms.
- Stand next to a chair and support your weight.
- Lift one leg and rest it on top of a chair.
- Stand up straight and lean backwards and forwards to loosen your back and spine.

The Slow Dance

The "slow dance" uses gravity and movement to increase comfort during birthing time. It is also easy to use other comfort measures while in this position, such as any of the relaxation techniques, breathing, counter-pressure, or hot/cold tools. This position can also be very emotionally supportive for the mother. It is usually done by rhythmically rocking back and forth, with or without music, as the mother puts her arms around the birth companion's neck and shoulders. The birth companion can apply counter pressure to any particular spot or simply wrap their arms around the mother's belly. She can rest her head on the companion's shoulder or neck if she prefers.

Kneeling

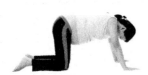

Kneeling can take the pressure off your back and help to relieve back discomfort. Importantly, it helps a baby rotate to the most favorable position: occiput anterior (OA). You may like to use these positions when you are in a surge or between surges.

- Hands and knees on the floor with pillows on the ground.
- Hands and knees on the bed.
- Kneel over a chair with a pillow for your head and knees.
- Pelvic Tilt Exercise helps reduce back discomfort in labor.
- Put your bottom in the air and head on a pillow *(best position for turning a posterior baby)*.
- Lay in a yoga 'child's pose' with your head on a pillow and legs tucked underneath.

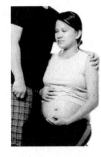

Sitting

Sitting in a chair or on an exercise ball is much better than sitting in a bed. As your feet are lower than your hip, which helps the pelvis to open. Sitting also helps the baby's decent. It also provides support so you can focus on your surges and rest between surges. Have your birth partner support you in your sitting position. It is also useful position for touch relaxation, light touch and counter pressure massages.

- Sit on an exercise ball, supported by your partner.
- Rocking chairs can be very relaxing and comforting *(rest your feet on a few pillows)*.
- Sit on a chair the wrong way around; with your front against the back support, with a pillow.
- Sit cross legged on the floor or bed.
- Sit on a recliner if available.
- Sit in the shower on a plastic chair.
- Sit in the bath with your knees up, while sitting on a waterproof pillow.
- Sitting on the toilet with a pillow for your head, can be useful to have a mental association with relaxing and releasing.

Squatting

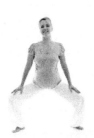

Squatting helps your baby ease down into your pelvis and opens the pelvis to provide more room for your baby. This position also uses gravity to help the baby decent. Your pelvis will open wider if your knees are **lower** than your hips. So, make sure your squatting isn't too deep and near the floor.

Squat against a wall for support or have an exercise ball behind you and have your partner support you in your squat with their arms under yours. Only squat as long as you are comfortable with, don't tire yourself out!

- Sit on an exercise ball with your legs wide apart like a squat and make sure the ball is pumped up so your hips are higher than your knees. This isn't a full squat, but works quite well and still beneficial.
- Squatting can be done on the bed or in the pool.
- See if the hospital bed has a squatting bar.

Moving Your Hips

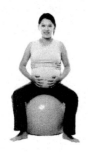

Remember to rock your hips backwards and forwards, side to side or in a circle to help your baby through your pelvis and to comfort yourself. You may recall these exercises in Unit 1. You'll be more likely to use these positions in labor if they are familiar to you while you are still pregnant.

Sit on an exercise ball and roll your hips backwards and forwards, side to side. Then roll your hips around in a circle, like doing the hula hoop. Next, sway your hips against a wall or partner for support. Then, sway side to side while holding on the handle of an open door.

Side Lying

When using a side lying position during labor, the mother will rest on one side, with her body slightly curled. The mother is able to reduce unnecessary muscular effort, which, in turn, lessens fatigue in a long labor and greatly increases her comfort level.

This position is very beneficial for the baby as well. It removes pressure from the uterus, kidneys, or other internal organs that can compress the umbilical cord. Side-lying, particularly on the left side, is often used in hospitals when the baby's heart rate decreases during surges.

During early birthing time, side-lying may not be the best choice as many of the other upright positions encourage speedier labor by using gravity to move the baby down through the pelvis. The side lying option can be particularly useful for a lengthy labor or when the mother is having difficulty maintaining adequate relaxation. While it is important to remain active in your birth, if you need to lie down and rest, then this is the best choice of position.

> Changing your position - sitting, kneeling, standing, lying down, getting on your hands and knees and walking, all help relieve discomfort and facilitate the birth by adding the benefits of gravity and changes in the shape of the pelvis. Swaying from side to side, rocking, or other rhythmic movements are both comforting and a great way to get the baby into a good position.

Active - Early Birthing   (1 - 4cm)

It is not necessary to be active for the whole time. Firstly you will wear yourself out! If you do need rest, it is better to sit upright or do side-lying. If you are having your surges at night, sleeping between surges is perfectly fine as your body is more relaxed and responsive if it is fully rested.

During surges:

Go to your special place and relax fully so you can focus on your surge breathing.

You may like to:

- Sit on a chair with your head against a pillow
- On all fours with your head resting against an exercise ball
- Relax in a bath or shower, sitting down
- Sit on a recliner with a pillow for your head

For this early part of the birthing are some tips:

- Upright or standing positions for childbirth use gravity to encourage surges to progress. They are among the best options for early labor and can help contractions to become regular and rhythmic.
- Walking is ideal for getting surges more regular and helps to progress this stage.
- Kneeling forwards over the ball takes the weight off your back and is great if you have back discomfort.
- Simply by sitting and rolling with the ball encourages rhythmic movement and pelvic mobility.

Active - Established Birthing (4 - 8cm)

During this time, your body is doing an amazing job of preparing for birth. By being active you are encouraging this process to move along quickly. At this stage, you may find that your surges are getting more intense and you may need some extra comfort measures. Choose active positions that expose your back for your partner to provide massage or relaxation techniques.

During surges:

- Remember deep relaxation is the key to your comfortable surges. The more relaxed you are, the easier they will be. It is important that you and your partner do all that you can to encourage the deepest level of relaxation.
- You may want to be active during your surge, or you simply may want to find the best position to relax and focus on your surge breathing.
- To bring additional comfort to a surge, lift your bottom and leaning forward with the surge.
- Some find it helpful to rock with each surge while leaning forwards and straightening up in between surges.
- If you feel it helps you cope, ask your birth partner or midwife to provide a counter pressure massage your back with each surge.
- If you get really tired and bed seems like the best place to be, use pillows or wedges to lie down on your side. Remember that surges are more intense in laying down positions, so you'll need to balance your need for rest with how you're coping.

Active - Transition (8-10cm)

It is the time that your body has the last two centimetres to go before your baby is ready to start its journey down to meet you. While it is true that some women find this time physically challenging with intense surges, it is more often a mental and hormonal issue rather than an increased physical demand on the body. The most important thing to remember is that this time is short and can be over in five to thirty minutes. The best thing about transition is that you should get a rest afterwards where surges stop for a short time. So hang in there, you have almost made it!

Being upright allows the **bones and ligaments of the pelvis to move and adjust** to ease the passage for the baby. This is especially true of the coccyx or tailbone, as it can move backwards during the last stages of labor, thus increasing the amount of space for the baby to move through the birth canal. This cannot happen if a woman is lying on her back. So be as upright as you can now for this last remaining bit.

BIRTHING - BEST POSITIONS

Squatting

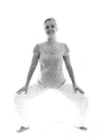

Squatting is the **most beneficial birth position** in that it opens the pelvis wide, shortens the birth path and uses gravity to encourage the baby to descend. This position is known to shorten the birthing phase of labor by helping the baby drop as far as possible without any conscious effort. It is the position that is most used by women worldwide, particularly in more remote and village births. Throughout early history, squatting when giving birth has been depicted often.

While squatting is certainly effective, it can also be tiring and will require a lot of preparation exercises prior to birth. If you can squat continuously for five minutes, most likely squatting will be an option for you. Although, it isn't necessary to maintain this position through the whole birthing phase, but rather to help the mother into this position during surges or when her body tells her this is what she needs.

A correct squatting position is achieved when the mother opens her legs and bends her hips, and brings her rear close to the floor *(but above her knees)* while keeping her feet flat on the floor or bed. This can be difficult for a mother as it requires balance and can be a strain on her leg muscles. For this reason, a birth companion or two may be enlisted for support.

Squat bar or with a birth partner

For a hospital birth, the mother may have access to a childbirth squat bar which is attached over the end of the bed. The mother squats above the bed while grasping the bar for support. If one isn't available, then a birth companion can support each leg while she squats. She can rest on the bed until the surge begins, and then resumes the squatting. The benefit to hospital staff with a squat bar is they have easy access to see how the birth is progressing.

A birth stool

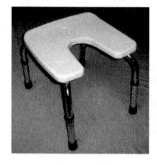

A birthing stool is a viable option to squatting. This is a short, u-shaped stool or chair. The mother sits upon it, which puts her body into a squatting position while supporting her weight. This has the benefit of squatting, but **doesn't put stress and pressure on her legs**. Check if your birthing facility has a birth stool, or bring your own in. Some obstetricians prefer not to encourage births on stools as they don't have a clear sight and access to the birth. However, this is your birth and your choice, so make your wishes clear.

Over a birth ball

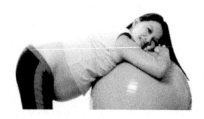

A woman kneels on the floor *(supported by cushions)* with her legs wide apart and bottom in the air. This is becoming a popular way to birth, as it has the benefit of a women being able to rest her head on the ball for the surge and stay in this comfortable position for the birth. As her legs and hips are wide apart and almost in a squatted position, she is using the benefits of a squat without the effort. Although the squat makes a better use of gravity, birthing over a ball is still a good choice. Medical staff encourages this option as they have an excellent view of how birth is progressing.

Birthing on all fours

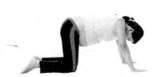

This is still an effective method of birthing and one that is particularly useful if the baby is in a challenging position or is a particularly large baby. The benefit of this position is that birthing is slowed down due to less utilization of gravity, but still in a natural and safe birthing position. If the baby is large, there is less pressure of the perineum, and there is less chance of tearing.

Birthing in water

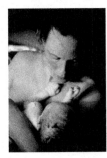

Often, women stretch their legs out to the edge of the bath or pool, so they can get a better grip and stability to birth. This movement inadvertently means they are lying almost on their backs when they give birth. As we know this is not the most effective position, even in water. It is important to make sure you feel supported in your chosen active birth position. Perhaps have a midwife hold your feet and your partner support you from behind or in the pool. Many positions can be done in water, so find out which one suits you.

Side lying (also good for epidurals)

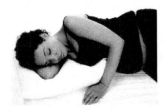

When using a side lying position during birthing, the mother will rest on one side, with her body slightly curled and one leg lifted up and supported. This birth position is particularly effective for maintaining relaxation and is very beneficial for the baby, as well. They remove pressure from the uterus, kidneys, or other internal organs that can compress the umbilical cord.

She will most likely need to **assist her body a little more** when compared to more squatting positions, as gravity is not in operation. However it is a good 'compromise' position if the mother is excessively tired. If she has had an epidural and isn't able to get into a more active position, then side lying is the better option than lying on her back or being in a semi reclined position. In side laying it is easier to use the 'Perfect Pushing for Intervention' and engage correct muscles when compared to birthing on her back.

COMFORT MEASURES FOR BIRTH

Creating the best birth environment

It is interesting to note that the optimal conditions for giving birth mirror the optimal conditions for conceiving a baby. During lovemaking, the woman's body produces high levels of oxytocin as long as she feels safe, private, warm and unobserved. The more relaxed and confident she is, the more enjoyable the experience will be.

Whether you choose to give birth at home, birthing center or in hospital, there are certain things that you can do to facilitate the most natural and comfortable birth. Here are a few basic guidelines,

- **Privacy:** A birthing mother should not feel observed. This includes using cameras, videos and foetal monitors as this can increase her levels of anxiety, inhibitions and an expectation to perform. Just think, how easy would it be for you to fall asleep knowing people are watching you?

  It is therefore not surprising that many women who go into hospital to give birth choose to spend a lot of time in the bathroom or the toilet where they can close or even lock the door and be left alone.

- **Safety:** If a woman feels anxious or scared, her body will not be able to birth effectively. Therefore, as far as possible, choose to give birth in a place where you feel safe and well cared for and aim to reduce all potential concerns and anxieties.

- **Quiet:** When a woman is in established labor, it is important that she is able to focus inwards and is not distracted by noises around her. Simply asking her a question can bring her out of her "zone" and disrupt the hormonal dance of labor. Even though she may appear to be "away with the fairies", she will still be able to hear everything around her and so any unnecessary or disruptive conversation may disturb her.

- **Low lights:** Bright lights are stimulating and can be intimidating, as they naturally increase the flow of adrenalin. In addition, a woman in a brightly lit room may feel more observed. A mother will feel calmer, safer and more private if the lights are dimmed.

- **Warmth:** The temperature is also important. If a mother gets cold, she will start to produce adrenalin, and will divert blood away from the uterus in order to maintain her body temperature.

'No Noise Rule' during a surge. Partners should stay as quiet as possible during a surge and everyone is to be silent to allow you to focus and work with your body.

Your best birth hospital environment

If you are having a home birth, then a factor for your choice usually lies in the comfort and confidence in birthing in your own home and surroundings. For mothers who choose a hospital of birth center birth, the object is to recreate this familiar feeling of comfort and 'own space'. Here are a few suggestions:

1. **Have your own duvet or blanket** - What does your duvet represent to you? Comfort, safety, warmth, privacy?

2. **Earplugs or earphones** - To block out any noise and so stay focused.

3. **Eye mask** - To make your space a little darker.

4. **Turn off lights and close curtains** - Switch on an angle poise lamp and turn it towards the wall to get a small amount of diffused light. Many midwives are happy to use a torch in a darkened room so that they can see what is happening without disturbing the mother. You can also bring in electric tea lights which give off a small candle-like light but without the flame. Aromatherapy and personal items can also be brought in.

5. **'Do not disturb' sign** - Place a sign outside the door asking not to be disturbed and for anyone to knock and then wait to be invited in.

6. **Cover up unnecessary equipment** - Throw a sheet or blanket over any medical/clinical equipment to help make your space more comforting and homely.

7. **Bring your own clothes to birth in** - Using hospital gowns make you feel like a patient not a parent. An oversized t-shirt is good.

8. **Ipod, tablet/phone** - With Birth Music and the Hypnobirthing Home Study Course CDs/recordings.

Relaxation is key to good births

The foundation stone to your successful hypnobirthing experience is a measure of how deeply you can relax during your birthing time. The Hypnobirthing Home Study Course teaches you how to relax at will, so when you need relaxation, **you will be able to call upon this natural state of being calm**

instantly. While the concept may be strange to begin with, it is entirely possible in a short space of time to transform your ability to relax at will.

Your needs and emotional state are going to vary a great deal throughout the birth; therefore it is useful to learn a wide range of comfort measures with your birth partner and have a "tool kit" that you can dip into at different times. In addition to your breathing, relaxation triggers and the Hypnobirthing Home Study Course recordings, there are many practical exercises and ways to prepare for a comfortable birth. Therefore, there are bound to be a few specific tools that will work well for you on the day.

Here are a few things to get started:

- What things make you feel calm and at ease?
- In what environments do you feel most happy?
- How do you know you are relaxed?
- Is it certain kinds of music, or a massage, soothing voices, aromatherapy smells,
- A bath, shower, meditation, prayer, chanting, a walk on a beach, or a swing in a hammock?

Make a list of those things and see what you can do to incorporate these into your birth.

RELAXATION - MIND, THOUGHTS AND ATTENTION

The Beginning: In early or pre labor you may wish to simply relax, practice relaxation breathing rhythmically and easily through your early surges. Close your eyes, and visualize either something very soothing and pleasant or the surges opening the cervix and pressing the baby downward. Perhaps put the birth music on to create the relaxation trigger. The more relaxed you are at this stage, the easier and more prepared you will be for the next stage of birth.

Your Special Place: Go to the special place you have practiced during your pregnancy. This might be the same or it might be different. Use **the trigger 1,2,3,4 ....release** to transport you to this place.

Your Internal Body: You might **visualize exactly what is happening** inside your body, the long muscles of the uterus reaching down to gently pull open the round muscles of the cervix, the surges massaging the baby, and the baby pressing down and opening the cervix.

Metaphor: Many women like to imagine a different scenario that matches the emotions and feelings of contractions. This could be the picture of experiencing yourself riding above your contractions, as if you are riding on the **crest of a wave** or are a sea gull above a stormy sea, soaring over, but still very much in touch with the surges.

Auditory Stimulus: Focusing on **sounds** such as your birth music, the soothing voice of your birth partner, a recording of various natural sounds *(surf, rain, a babbling brook),* repeating rhythms, or other sounds. Many women naturally use sounds to help them through surges. When a woman opens her throat, vocalises, hums, moans, or groans through a surge, she is also opening her birth canal. It can be a really powerful way of releasing tension and relaxing the body.

The next time you get a practice surge (Braxton Hicks), rehearse all these relaxation techniques, so they will be second nature to you when you need them most.

USING YOUR BODY FOR A COMFORTABLE BIRTH

The Power of Touch - Endorphin Release

Massage and touch stimulates endorphin release *(the body's natural painkillers)* to help reduce sensations. Endorphins are manufactured by our bodies in response to strong sensations and act as a natural way to regulate sensations. Endorphins are released by the descending nerve fibers or nerves which travel down the spinal cord from the brain.

The release of endorphins by the nerves inhibits some or all of the pain messages going up to the brain. For many women, endorphins will also positively alter the memory of their birth experience and in some cases induce an amnesic, dreamy effect. Endorphins can therefore empower women and provide a positive memory and experience associated with their birthing time.

Massages release endorphins

Massage not only feels good. Research shows it reduces the heart rate, lowers blood pressure, increases blood circulation and lymph flow, relaxes muscles, and improves range of emotion and most importantly for birthing increases endorphins. During massage, large amounts of these **endorphins are released into the bloodstream.** This explains the feeling you may have afterwards of being slightly groggy and lightheaded, but with a calm sense of wellbeing.

> *The mind, which before massage is in a perturbed, restless, vacillating, and even despondent state, becomes calm, quiet, peaceful, and subdued after massage. In fact, the wearied and worried mind has been converted into a mind restful, placid, and refreshed.*
> Dr. Dowse 1887

LIGHT TOUCH MASSAGE MAXIMIZES ENDORPHINS

Gently touch your neck lightly with your fingers, stroke your ears, and feel your head ever so lightly. Did you notice a tingly sensation? Did you even get bumps on your arms? Felt good? Well, you just released some endorphins into your system. The lighter, softer, and gentler the massage, the more it releases which has the ability to release lots of the sensation numbing hormones. Many women in birthing just love this type of light tickly touch massage. A woman in birthing is at times too sensitive for deep massage to feel relaxing, and so the light touch massage works a treat.

Light touch massage technique

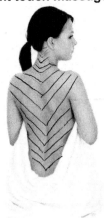 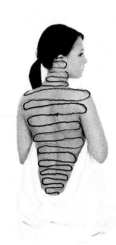

Figure 1 – V shapes with your finger tips   Figure 2 - S shapes with your finger tips

Kneel over a birthing ball or sitting sideways on a chair with your back facing your partner.

V shapes. Then ever so lightly with the very **tips of your fingers** gently form a series of V shapes from the base of her spine up her neck, ears and down her arms. **Repeat three times.**

S Shapes. Then form a series of S shapes from the base of her spine up again to her neck, ears and down her arms. **Repeat three times**.

During her birthing, women may either love it or hate this technique. As a partner, it is important to pick up on her cues as to whether she is benefiting from it or not. I do suggest that partners practice this every night along with a good foot massage!

See our website for a free instructional video on this technique, or download the free App on iTunes and Android

COUNTER BACK PRESSURE MASSAGE

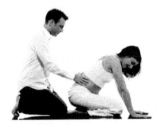 Another helpful form of massage for birth is **firm pressure used particularly over the lower back or sacrum during surges.** Counter pressure is an effective way to manage the sensations during a surge. It is a particularly useful strategy for feelings of intense pressure in the back or other area-specific discomfort. For many women, this counter pressure can make a big difference.

Counter pressure technique

This technique also called **sacral pressure** is especially helpful for easing any discomfort in the back during surges. Your partner presses the heel of both hands on the sacral area of your lower back and simply holds it there for the duration of the surge. During labor, you may be surprised at how much pressure you want, so make sure you give that feedback to your partner.

The exact spot for applying pressure **varies from woman to woman, and changes during her birthing time**. Thus it is difficult to know in advance which spot will be best. You may need a surprising amount of pressure, which may be very tiring for your partner after even a few minutes. It is worth the effort, though, as the relief and comfort it brings can be immense. Your partner can take turns with another support person to allow him or her to take a rest.

Tennis ball massage technique

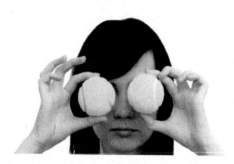

Counter pressure massage can be extremely tiring, and this is a way to save your muscles! This simple massager that you can make, will take away tension from your lower back and is so easy but effective to use. All you need it two tennis balls and some tights or socks. See this great step by step video to make yours 'Amazing back massager for pregnant women' http://www.youtube.com/watch?v=I-nhQsB9B_c Women may like using the tennis ball massager on themselves, by leaning up against a wall with the tennis balls and finding the right spot to massage. *See our website for a free instructional video on this technique, or download the free App on iTunes and Android*

Shaking things ups

What is the first thing you do if you have banged or hurt yourself? Instinctively, you rub it vigorously, which often makes it feel better.

"Shaking things up" simply involves standing behind the mother as she leans on a chair or kneels over the ball or bed. Using both hands, vigorously rub the mother's back, hips, bottom, thighs, and legs! As an alternative, use a '**Rebozo**' is a great way to give your arms a rest. Simply put a Rebozo or something like a thick sarong or small sheet over the mother's bottom and then rub. There are more benefits from a Rebozo to use in labor to get your baby into the best possible birth position.

This should be done between surges and at times when she needs a boost or a change. It is especially useful if she has had an adrenalin blip and needs to get back into the "zone" .This may be due to her waters releasing and the next surge being very intense, or it may be after a new person has come on the scene or after moving to another place to have her baby. There are many benefits of using this technique. It helps with:

- Releasing adrenalin.
- Releasing lactic acid.
- Releasing tension in the vital areas around the cervix and pelvis.
- Increasing blood flow to the birthing area.
- Helping the mother release tension all over.
- Making her laugh!

Warm water

What is one of the first things you like to do after a long, hard day, or when you are feeling a bit under the weather? For many, it is taking a long, warm soak in the bath. This, of course, is especially wonderful during birthing. As soon as you enter warm water, your body instinctively relaxes, which makes the surges more manageable.

The use of water as a method of managing surges was pioneered in the 1970s by Michel Odent, and has increased in popularity in recent years, with most maternity units having water birth facilities. For women choosing to have their babies at home, it has become even easier and more affordable to buy or rent a pool.

Research into water births has shown that they are extremely safe and in many ways help women to have more instinctive and drug-free births.

According to Janet Balaskas in her book on water births, the benefits to a woman in birthing are that being in water:

- Increases privacy
- Provides significant reduction in sensations
- Reduces the need for drugs and interventions
- Encourages a woman's sense of control in her birth
- Facilitates mobility and enables optimal positions for an active birth
- Speeds up birthing time
- Promotes relaxation and conserves energy
- Helps to reduce perineal tears
- Encourages an easier birth for the mother and a gentler welcome for the baby

It is important not to get too hung up on wanting a "water birth" - for some women, when it actually comes to birthing their babies; they really want to get out of the water, and want to be on dry land. See the use of water as a comfort measure, rather than as a predetermined outcome.

In addition, some facilities permit you to labor in water, but won't allow you to birth in water. Midwives and obstetricians need to have special training to facilitate a water birth and you may not have one of these caregivers when you birth. Also, some obstetricians prefer not deliver in water and are concerned with a small risk of infection if the bath/pool is not properly cleaned before use.

Make the most of a water birth

1. **Leave settling in the pool as long as you can**. In some hospitals, the guidelines are that you should wait until you are five centimetres dilated. However, if you are not choosing to have vaginal exams and do not want to know how many centimetres you are, then simply hold off until you really feel like you need some additional support. The most important factor is that your surges are regular and increasing in intensity. Women have gone from three centimetres to fully dilated in a very short amount of time, but the key was that their surges were strong and regular.

2. **Do not stay in the pool continually for more than two hours**. It is a good idea to get out, have a walk around, go to the toilet, let your skin breathe and have a change of scenery.

3. **Keep the water at a temperature that is comfortable for you during the birth**. Women often like the water to be a lower temperature than a normal bath. However, it is recommended that the water is approximately thirty-five to thirty-seven degrees, especially for around the time the baby is born. If you are at home, make sure you are familiar with putting the pool up and knowing how long it takes to fill up, remembering to turn on the immersion heater/boiler.

Warm shower will work wonders

If you do not have a birth pool or bath, you can still benefit from taking a long, warm shower. In the shower, lean against the wall or sit on a towel-covered stool so that you can rest. Direct the spray where it helps most - maybe on your lower back or on your lower abdomen. If you are in the bath, cover your tummy with a warm, wet hand towel. It will stop your tummy from getting cold!

Hot packs

Gentle heat encourages blood flow and relaxation of muscles, which of course is beneficial during the birthing time. When heat is applied to the low abdomen, back, groin or perineum, it can be very soothing. There are lots of things you can use, such as a hot-water bottle, or hot compresses made up of washcloths or small towels soaked in hot water, wrung out, and quickly applied wherever you need them. As they cool, they should be replaced.

As an alternative, try a hot pack from camping store or chemist. You can have the ones that are wheat or gel packs that you heat in the microwave or if you don't want to leave the room, a Chemical reaction hot pack that you use in hiking to heat your hands is just the right temperature for skin and keep warm for a long time. Simply squeeze the pack to create heat.

Cold packs

On the other hand, applying a cold pack can also provide a great deal of relief, especially as your body is "hotting up" in the established birthing time. A cold pack can be anything - an ice bag, a rubber glove filled with crushed ice, a bag of frozen peas, "instant" cold packs, or frozen gel packs. Placed on the forehead, or a cold pack placed on the lower back during labor or on the *perineum immediately after birth to reduce pain and swelling.* For cold packs to bring comfort, however, you must be feeling comfortably warm. If you are feeling chilled, a cold pack should not be used.

Use common sense in deciding how hot or cold the compresses should be. When in your birthing time, you might easily tolerate compresses so hot or cold that they could damage your skin. Cover these with a towel to make sure that your skin is protected. You should not use a cold compress on the perineum for more than ten to fifteen minutes, as it will decrease the blood flow to the area and so slow down healing.

Aromatherapy oils

Another useful comfort measure in childbirth is the use of aromatherapy oils. You cannot take a candle burner into hospital, then you can now buy electric oil burners that plug into a normal socket, or you can buy a terracotta ring that you put on top of an electric light bulb.

Some of the most common and recommended oils for use during the labor are **lavender, neroli, marjoram, rose,** and **clary sage**. Clary sage is to encourage labor and stimulate surges if things are very slow to start or have really slowed down during labor. However, it is advised to avoid clary sage during pregnancy.

If you like the smell of oils, then burn them at the same time you are listening to your birth music; as you will make the subconscious connection with the oils and relaxation, which will be triggered when you smell the oils during the birth.

Beverages

What is important is that you continue to take in liquids throughout the birthing process. Remember to **bring a straw** so that you can drink in any position you happen to be in. During your birthing, you usually can drink water, herbal tea or clear apple juice, or suck on ice. Hourly trips to the bathroom to urinate will increase your comfort during surges as it takes away any pressure around the bladder and makes more room for the baby to descend down into the birth canal. If you have a very dry mouth, you can suck on ice cubes, a lollipop, or glucose tablets.

Homeopathy

Some women just love homeopathic remedies for many are invaluable during birthing and will support and promote the physiological and mental process without any harmful side effects. It usually works best if your partner takes responsibility for offering you any remedies that you may need. This way, you can focus on the birthing. You can also consult a homeopath if you would like to put together a homeopathic labor kit that is specifically relevant to you. Alternatively many health food stores sell pre made labor kits, pregnancy, birth, and after homeopathic remedies.

Pain Gate Theory

Melzak and Wall proposed the 'Gate Theory' in 1965, and it remains the most respected theory of pain perception. They showed that pain impulses could be overridden and the perception of pain could be altered. It is a very personal experience and highly influenced by circumstances and interpretation. Pain occurs when specialized nerve receptors are stimulated and messages are passed from the nervous system to the brain *(dorsal horn)* where they are interpreted as pain.

The brain *(dorsal horn)* is responsible for passing on information which can be interpreted as pain. This area is referred to as the 'gate' as it prevents the brain from receiving too much information too quickly. Therefore, pain messages are prioritized and skin nerves signals are registered and the nerve fiber messages are lost. Our body has designed this process to protect us from immediate harm. It is much more dangerous for us to ignore our hand in fire for example, than for us to focus our attention on a backache.

There are two kinds of nerve fibers.

- **Nerve fibers** sense pain such as sharp and aching feelings.
- **Skin nerves** which carry senses of touch, heat, cold, numb and pressure. These are faster, and also have **priority** which effectively blocks out the pain messages from the nerve fibers to the brain and closes the gate.

Think of the skin sensations as an express train, and the aches and pains of muscles and bones, etc., as a slow train. The tracks are merging into one; there is a signal box ahead, which has a red light to the slow train and green light to the express train. Therefore it is express train (skin sensations) that makes it to the brain for interpretation.

Labor TENS machine and how it works

TENS is widely used around the world for a reducing discomfort and is now used in the birthing time. It is based on the 'Pain Gate Theory' and a small electrical device delivers electrical impulses across the skin. The device is connected by wires to sticky pad electrodes, which are placed on the skin in the area of the pain. This allows a small, low-intensity electric charge to be passed across the area. Impulses from the Labor TENS machine pass along nerve fibers to the brain and receive priority, by sending out a chemical blocker to 'close the gate' to pain. Labor TENS sensations are felt in the brain effectively overriding pain messages.

Unlike many pain-relieving drugs, TENS isn't addictive and seems to have few side-effects. Most people can use a TENS machine, but it's not suitable for:

- Epileptics
- Those with pacemakers and certain other types of heart disease
- Unknown causes of pain

TENS machines are not usually available in birthing units or hospitals and if you choose to use these, they will need to be purchased or hired in advance.

It has been found that strong skin sensations have priority going to the brain, and these sensations do not necessary mean pain. The TENS machine uses comfortable skin eclectic pluses which are effective in stopping painful body messages being sent.

Disadvantages of labor TENS

- The buzzing and pulsating sensations can distract from focusing on your surge breathing. Hypnobirthing Home Study Course recording 'Anesthesia for Birthing' is usually more effective, particularly if practiced regularly.
- Bathing or showering is not possible with a TENS machine.
- Challenge to do other techniques such a light touch or counter pressure massage when electrodes attached.

PAIN FREE BIRTHING IS POSSIBLE

'Anesthesia for Easy Birthing' – Hypnobirthing Home Study Course Mp3/Cd

This track teaches powerful pain management strategies while being completely relaxed and calm. It uses a **combination of deep relaxation Hypnosis and the 'Pain Gate Theory' to create a powerful anesthetised feeling in your hand.** This cold, numb feeling is **transferred** to another part of your body if you should feel discomfort when in your birthing time.

It is not essential for you to learn this tool, as many Hypnobirthing Hub mother's find the other tools and techniques more than enough to have a pain-free and easy birth. However, women have found this technique of most benefit for difficult position births such as posterior, lengthy births and those needing something extra to keep the epidural at bay.

We know that your brain will prioritize the nerve signals of cold and numb in favor of nerve signals of sharpness or achiness when you are in your birthing time, so we use these to our advantage and create **cold numb anesthetised effect with our mind**. Our mind and body are connected and under hypnosis we actually start to feel that our body is feeling numb and anesthetised. In this way, the more painful sensations of sharp feelings, sometimes found in labor are significantly reduced or even eliminated.

Think of the express train being skin sensations of numb and cold. We create these with our mind and the slow train being the sharp or achiness birthing pains. The skin sensations have priority and stop the pain messages from getting through.

It is a wonderful and very powerful sensation. In fact, many mothers have found this to be such an incredibly effective comfort measure in birthing. This is because you are combining the effects of deep relaxation, comfort and numbness to birth in the most comfortable way possible.

Creating Anesthesia with Hypnosis is not new

Remember back to the section on hypnosis and its history? You will recall how hypnosis was used in child birth, and before medical drugs. Hypnosis was used in operations with pain free results. Even today, if a person is allergic to anesthetics, the patient will work with a hypnotherapist over a month, to create deep anesthesia in the body. In time, the patient is able to be operated on fully awake, yet relaxed and comfortable. The same anesthesia comfort is possible for you at your birthing as well.

The key is to believe that it will happen and secondly to practice until the trigger and lack of sensation is automatic.

 How the natural Anesthesia trigger works

If you choose to listen to the Hypnobirthing Home Study Course recording **Creating Anesthesia for Birthing**: you will be creating anesthesia triggers. It will be your hand that will start to feel numb and anesthetised. Then you will have the ability to transfer that numb feeling to any part of your body that you need when you are in your birthing time. These triggers are similar to relaxation trigger 1,2,3,4 ....relax; where you have already practiced gaining instant deep relaxation.

To aid memory and familiarity; most of the Hypnobirthing tools start with 1,2,3,4....

Relaxation Breathing	1,2,3,4.... (out 1,2,3,4,5,6,7,8)
Relaxation Trigger	1,2,3,4 .... relax (also with hand on shoulder)
Relaxation Trigger	1,2,3,4 .... relax (transported to special place)
Quick Release Trigger	1,2,3,4 .... release

The Anesthesia triggers follows similar patterns:

Hand becoming numb	(1,2,3,4) ....numb
Transferring anesthesia	1,2,3,4 .... release

The release triggers

The Quick release trigger (1,2,3,4....release) follows the same pattern as the Anesthesia release trigger (1,2,3,4 ....release). As you become familiar with using the emotional release trigger to release the emotions from your mind and your body, you will find it very easy to use the same concept to release and transfer the feeling of numbness in your hand to another part of your body.

Practice, practice, practice

In order to be most effective on the day, you need to be able to create the numbing sensation in your hand and be able to transfer this feeling to another part of your body. Some people will easily feel numb tingly sensations in their hand from the very first listening. Others may take some time, as this is the most advanced hypnobirthing tool and, as such, requires the most practice to be effective. Keep at it - you will get it!

Gauge your progress by using the triggers whenever you have some discomfort in your body during your pregnancy. Many mothers and fathers to be have benefited from using this tool and found relief from headaches, backaches and other ailments. It is a very powerful tool to use, and you owe it to yourself and your baby to practice this tool until you can easily create the numbing sensation and transfer this to another part of your body.

Tip: Sit up in chair (not lying down in bed and sleeping) with your hands apart and keep them apart for the session. Just before you start, place an ice pack on your hands for a few seconds. This will remind you of the cold numbing sensation that you are going to recreate in your mind.

Sterile water injections (SWI)

The concept behind the development of sterile water injections for **back pain in labor** is 'Pain Gate Theory'. We know that the skin receptors have priority over nerve receptors that relay the sensations to our brain of dull aching pain in our back. So, when a woman has intractable back pain, often because of the baby being in the posterior position, then the water injections into her skin may be useful.

If a woman has the water injections into her skin, it stings for about thirty seconds, similar to a wasp sting. That sting switches on the skin nerve fibers and these signals from the skin come racing up to the gate, the traffic controlling chemicals recognize an immediate threat, **close the gate to the back ache messages and let the quick skin nerve message through**. The result: the back pain is stopped in its tracks and the woman no longer feels that internal sensation. That effect lasts for about 90 minutes.

How effective and safe are sterile water injections?

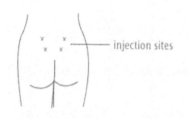
injection sites

They are very effective for the majority of women. The pain level of the back pain has to be a high enough level, so that the wasp like sting is worth it. On a 0-10 score, with ten being the worst pain imaginable, the pain level has to be about a seven or above.

It is a completely **natural treatment with no side effects** and will not harm the mother or baby. Check with your hospital or birthing center to see if they provide Sterile Water Injections.

> ⓘ   SWI are an excellent alternative for relief of back pain in labor, although SWI will not provide pain relief from surge sensations.

YOUR BIRTH PLAN

Too often couples come away from their birthing experiences expressing their disappointment with phrases such as "Oh, well," "The next time..." or "If only they hadn't..."

If you and your birthing partner have a clear vision of what you believe will allow you to have the most natural, gentle, and satisfying birthing for you and your baby, then you will need a birth plan to effectively communicate your birth vision. By consciously thinking about all aspects of labor and birth, you are more likely to achieve the birth you wish for and look back on your experience in a positive light knowing that you were fully informed. In the unlikely event that your birth required medical intervention, you will be confident in knowing that you did all you could to have a natural birth.

Yet sometimes circumstances are out of our control. This empowered thinking is proven to reduce the likelihood of post-natal depression. It is the mothers who felt a lack of choice and control at their birthing time; rather than the actual disappointing event that is a trigger of a post-natal depression period.

In the absence of your plan in hand, medical staff will follow their usual and routine procedures and assume that you wish to have your birth 'managed' by the medical staff. Most midwives in the labor and birthing area are there because they feel a strong dedication to being part of the birthing miracle and are more than willing to assist you in making your birthing the special event that you have planned.

Hypnobirthing is increasing in popularity and is usually very well regarded by midwives and obstetricians. Ask specifically for a midwife who knows and supports hypnobirthing. If this is not possible, alternatively request a midwife who is partial to natural births.

Download a copy of the birth plan to create your own birth choices at:
www.hypnobirthinghub.com/resourses

 Midwives Thoughts

"I like birth plans for a few reasons:

1. They show the women that they do have a choice in things … a lot of women still assume they have to do whatever they're told.

2. My experience is that if the woman states what she wants verbally it is easier for others to ignore it, or it gets lost in change of staff whereas if it's written it's given more respect.

3. If a copy of the birth plan is in the woman's notes prior to birth and the staff are able to read it before the woman comes in; sometimes it results in the most appropriate midwife being able to care for that woman. That is, midwives who aren't comfortable with the birth plan asking for someone else to care for the woman. (I know this doesn't reflect well on midwives as far as giving woman centered care, but the woman benefits if she ends up with a different midwife who will respect her wishes)." **Molly Jones, California, US**

Select a supportive caregiver

To ensure that your birthing does not needlessly turn into a "medical incident," you will need to select medical caregivers who will listen to you and respect your philosophy and your wishes. Talking with your doctor or midwife should take place early in your pregnancy and not simply left to a chance conversation later on.

If you've selected a clinic or association that has a rotating staff of doctors or midwives, anyone of whom could be attending your birth. Then ask that each be given a copy of your birth plan and suggest that a copy be put into your folder at the desk in the labor wing of the hospital or birthing centre.

Bring copies to the birth

Become a 'sales person' for your birth plan. If you are seeing a midwife for the first time, it is the **role of the birth partner** to sit down with her and go through the plan together, BEFORE most of your birthing time has begun. In this way, misunderstandings are cleared up early. Have another copy with you in your birthing room, so it can be referred to easily. Remember, even if you're birthing with your private obstetrician, you most likely will be meeting a new midwife who will be with you for the labor and birth. Her role is to provide telephone updates to your obstetrician, be given instructions and advise him or her when to attend the birth. Therefore, it is even more important that you clear up any concerns through your birth plan early.

If you plan to have a home birth, you will want to ensure your midwife and anyone else who will be present has a copy of the plan. Guests should know that you have a plan in place and this is not the time to relate stories of the progress of their own births or attempt to give you advice. **You are the stars, directors, and producers in this birth**.

Mother's Thoughts

'I had a private obstetrician for my first birth and he seemed really supportive of my Hypnobirth and kept a copy of my birth plan. But I forgot that on the day, I would have a midwife I hadn't met before and we didn't spend the time taking her through our birth plan (big mistake!). When I got my 'urge' I was ready to birth. I was in a really comfortable position; kneeling with arms over a birth ball and confident that I would birth well here.

My midwife said, 'Now on the bed, lie on your side, leg up.....your doctor delivers in this position.' She was adamant and I reluctantly complied. And with that, I lost all my confidence in my birthing body. It was a much more difficult birth, requiring an episiotomy and strong pushing. Later when I spoke to my doctor and expressed my annoyance, he said 'I am happy for you to birth in whatever position you chose. I was surprised when I came in for the birth that you were on the bed, I assumed you changed your mind… but hey, I delivered in that position, as I supported whatever you wanted.' **Catherine Johnstone, Sydney Australia**

Create a friendly tone in your plan

In writing your plan, you will want to keep in mind that your intent is not to "take on" your medical caregivers or practices that are currently in effect in the hospital or centre. Word your plan in such a way that it does not become an adversarial document of demands. You will want to assure staff that they will have your full cooperation should a medical necessity arise. Remember they are there to help you have a great birth experience and have the medical experience and knowledge to make that happen for you.

I may need to change my plan

If anything happens at your birth that may require a change of plan, remember the principle of being calm, relaxed and in control. Take a quick 'Relaxation breath' and remember to use your 'BRAIN'.

USE YOUR BRAIN FOR A CHANGE OF PLANS

Ask the Questions

- Is my partner in danger?
- Is the baby in danger?

If the answer is **NO**……. Then we would like to take some time for considering any change to our plan. Could we take about this again in an hour?

If the answer is **YES**….. Then ask the following;

Think BRAIN

B Benefits

R Risks

A Alternative

I Intuition

N Nothing (at least for a while)

You will know from the tone and the word choice of the medical staff to gauge how urgent the situation is. In this instance, be thankful for the expertise of our great medical system. The staff will guide you on what is the best approach in a medical emergency situation.

YOUR OPTIONS ...YOUR BIRTH PLAN

Overview of your birth

- Plans to have a natural birth
- Minimal intervention
- Hypnobirthing
- Specific to you? (VBAC? Medical concerns?)

Who is at your birth?

Specify who you plan on having with you during your birthing time

- your partner
- your children
- your doula or friend

What is your birthing environment?

- lighting
- temperature
- level of noise
- privacy
- use of shower/bath
- comfort measures: such as heat packs, massage, Homeopathy, Hypnobirthing Mp3s/CDs, aromatherapy and music
- What will make it special and feel 'homely' for you?

Movement in birthing?

- Birth Ball
- Exercise Mat
- Active Birth positions
- Freedom to move around and outside facility

Posterior or difficult position procedures?

- Positional changes to help move baby; such as hands and knees or Rebozo
- Hypnobirthing visualization and relaxation techniques
- Natural methods before intervention

Monitoring and vaginal exams?

- Doppler only (portable)
- Intermittent monitoring
- Continuous Electronic Foetal Monitoring (usually the mother needs to lie down and be attached to the monitor)
- Vaginal examinations to assess how far you are dilated (allow unlimited or only when you wish?)

Augmentation of labor (speeding up)?

- Natural methods of augmentation
- Releasing your membranes early
- Syntocinon only if absolutely necessary

Comfort measures in labor?

- Discussion of 'pain'?
- The use of natural comfort measures

- Hypnobirthing breathing and relaxation
- The use of gas to reduce discomfort
- Suggesting or administering pain relieving medication
- Suggesting or administering an epidural

Birthing positions? Available facilities?

- Birth Stool
- Birthing Ball
- Birth in bath/pool
- Birth in squatting position/on a squat bar
- Birth over an birthing ball

When the baby is being born?

- Natural comfort measures, such as heat packs or warm water on the perineum
- You or your partner/significant other to receive the baby (first to hold)
- Episiotomy?
- A mirror to view progress

Cutting your baby's cord?

- You cutting the cord or your partner/significant other cutting the cord
- Allow the cord to stop pulsating before being cut
- Cut the cord immediately
- Cord Blood collection
- Lotus birth (no cutting of cord, cord and placenta attached to baby detaches a week later)

Delivery of the placenta?

- Natural delivery with no timeframe
- Natural delivery if under 1hr of delivery
- Administering Syntocinon/Pitocin before the cord is cut
- Administering Syntocinon/Pitocin after the cord has stopped pulsating
- Administering Syntocinon/Pitocin only if there is signs of hemorrhaging

Immediately after your baby is born?

- Immediate skin-to-skin contact to allow bonding (no wiping of baby)
- Wiping baby first before skin-to-skin contact
- Breastfeeding support
- Weighing/measuring/ other routine
- Giving needles/heel pricks
- Bathing and dressing your baby
- Partner to stay with the baby if separated from mother

Vaccination and injections for baby?
- Oral vitamin K
- Injection of vitamin K
- Hepatitis B immediately at birth
- Hepatitis B a few days after birth or at GP surgery
- No vaccinations or injections

Other considerations

- How to discuss changes of plans with you and your partner
- Caesarean birth
- Special needs baby
- Your personal or religious beliefs

- Anything else you wish to put in to make this birth special

 Mother's Thoughts

"I decided to be pro-active and take control of my birthing experience. Accepting that I had to have a caesarean this time around didn't mean that I had to leave all the decisions in the hands of the doctors. I was actually going to make this happen! Everyone had been briefed as to what was in my birth plan and how I was going to contribute. "Okay, are you ready, here comes the head and the shoulders, now reach down." I reached down and linked my thumb and fingers around my baby's shoulders and lifted him onto my chest. The nurse had removed my hospital gown and my baby and I lay together (skin touching) for the first time. He was so soft and flexible and curled straight back into a little ball. As he lay on my chest, the warmth in my heart was unbelievable; everything seemed so surreal and wonderful!

For the women having caesarean births or other types of interventions without choice, it is important that they too know they can still take control of their situation and feel a part of 'bringing their baby into the world'. **Belinda Jefferies, Adelaide, Australia**

BIRTH PREFERENCES EXAMPLE

Our names are **Sarah Smith & Joe Bloggs**

We like to be called **Sarah** and **Joe**

Attending our birth: **Sally Smith (sister)**

Other notes: **Hypnobirthing**

We have chosen hypnobirthing, as our method to have a **natural childbirth without unnecessary interventions.** We have been trained in this child birth education method and are aware of our birth options.

We have given careful consideration to each specific request in our plan, and we feel that it represents our wishes at this time. We realise that as birthing ensues, we may choose to change our thinking and wish to feel free to do so.

We're looking forward to a normal pregnancy and birth and understand that these choices presume that this will be the case. Should a special circumstance arise that could cause us to deviate from our planned natural birth, we trust that you will provide us with a clear explanation of the special circumstance, the medical need for any procedure you may anticipate, and what options might be available. In such an event, please know that you will have our complete cooperation after we have had an explanation of the medical need and have had the opportunity to discuss the decision between ourselves.

In the absence of any special circumstance, we ask that the following requests be honoured. Thank you in advance for helping us obtain our wish for a joyous, memorable, and most satisfying natural birth.

Please make this information known to any other doctors, or midwives who may be attending the birth.

<signature>

<name>

Pre Admission

We request:

- ☐ To consider inducement only if onset of labor is unusually delayed and if there is medical urgency. Please perform an ultrasound to assess the health of the placenta and level of amniotic fluid.

- ☐ To use only natural means of inducement first, then moving to sweeping of the membranes. I would request two attempts before progressing to a hospital induction.

- ☐ If a hospital induction is required; and if prostaglandin gels are given; I request to return home to start labor in my own time.

- ☐ Only rupturing the membrane if medically required, then to return home to start labor on own time.

- ☐ Please give other inductions methods ample opportunity to work, with the pitocin/syntocinon drip as a last resort.

- ☐ If pitocin/syntocinon is medically required, please administer a very low dose, to be increased gradually and slowly and administered only after I reach 3-5cm dilation until labor is established. Then stop the dose to attempt the continued labor without artificial oxytocin.

- ☐ If membranes have been ruptured, naturally or artificially, please allow twenty-four hours before intervention. Please provide antibiotics rather than an induction.

Admission

We request:

- ☐ To return home until labor progresses further if less than four centimetres dilated.

- ☐ To have our birthing room with subdued lighting and drawn drapes for both labor and birthing.

- ☐ To have the following persons present during my birthing:
  - ○ partner
  - ○ relative
  - ○ other birthing companion
  - ○ labor support person

- ☐ To decline discussion on pain tolerance and levels

- ☐ No calls relayed--message only.

- ☐ Other requests:_____

ESTABLISHED BIRTHING (1ST STAGE OF LABOR)

We request:

Staff

- ☐ The patience and understanding of medical caregivers to refrain from any practice or procedure that could unnecessarily stand in the way of our having the most natural birth possible.

- ☐ Be allocated caregivers who support hypnobirthing or natural births.

- ☐ To allow labor to take its natural course without references to "moving things along." Please don't look at the clock.

- ☐ To be fully apprised and consulted before the introduction of <u>any</u> medical procedure. Please speak to my birth partner initially.

- ☐ Quiet and peace in a contraction, no talking please.

Comfort measures

- ☐ We ask that staff honour need for quiet and refrain from references to "pain", "hurt", or any offer of medication unless requested. In the event that I request pain relief, I would prefer to use gas/air before an epidural. I do not wish to use Pethidine.

- ☐ I plan to use hypnobirthing techniques for comfort measure, such as active birth positions and movement, massage, water, breathing, relaxation, visualization, heat/cold.

- ☐ Partner/birthing companion and other labor support person present at all times.

- ☐ To take fluids and light foods

- ☐ To take nutritional snacking if labor is prolonged.

- ☐ Freedom of choice to move (or not to move) during labor.

- ☐ To change positions and assume labor positions of choice.

- ☐ To enjoy labor tub or shower prior to rupturing of membranes.

- ☐ To have the use of a birthing ball if one is available.

- ☐ To have access to a birthing stool

Instruments/intervention

- ☐ To be free of blood pressure cuff between readings.

- ☐ In the absence of a medical necessity, only intermittent monitoring of baby's heart with fetoscope/doppler or manual use of EFM.

- ☐ No internal monitoring in the absence of foetal distress. To confirm distress, please perform a Fetal Lactate Sample.

- ☐ No internal electronic monitoring, as infection could be passed to the baby via the puncture site of an electrode clip on the scalp.

- ☐ Minimal number of vaginal exams, within reason, during the labor until the 'Foetal Expulsion Reflex' (urge).

- ☐ To use natural oxytocin stimulation in the event of a stalled or slow labor, nipple or clitoral stimulation and to be accorded the uninterrupted privacy to do so.

- ☐ No augmentation of labor without discussion and explanation of need.

☐   Other requests:_____

DURING BIRTHING OF OUR BABY (2ND STAGE)

We request:

☐   The patience and understanding of medical caregivers to refrain from any practice or procedure that could unnecessarily stand in the way of our having the most natural birth possible.

☐   To have the lights dimmed for birthing. If it is daylight, to access only natural light.

☐   To remain in tub for water birthing, if available.

☐   To allow natural birthing instincts (foetal expulsion reflex) to facilitate the descent of the baby, as much as possible, with mother-directed birth breathing down until crowning takes place.

☐   Use of hypnobirthing birth breathing techniques without staff prompts

☐   To birth in an atmosphere of gentle encouragement during the final birthing phase without coaching". Please calm, low tones, free of "pushing" prompts.

☐   To assume a birthing position of choice that will least likely require an episiotomy.

o   Use of birthing stool

o   Use of squatting bar on bed if available

o   Support with squatting during birthing

o   Leaning over a birth ball

☐   Oil and hot compresses to avoid episiotomy.

☐   Episiotomy only if necessary and only after consultation.

☐   Use of (topical) anaesthetic for episiotomy.

☐   Use of suctioning device rather than forceps if assistance is medically necessary.

☐   Use of mirror to enable me to see crowning and birth.

☐   To touch my baby's head at crowning.

☐   To discover the sex of the baby on my own.

☐   To have our other children present [ ] during [ ] shortly after birth.

☐   Mother [ ] Father [ ] other birth companion [ ] to help "receive" the baby if at all possible.

☐   To have the baby hear our voices first.

☐   Father or birth partner to remain with baby in the event of a surgical procedure.

NATURAL THIRD STAGE

☐   Father/birth partner to cut cord

☐   Delay cord clamping and cutting until after pulsation has ceased

☐   Allow up to an hour if necessary for natural placenta delivery.

☐   Immediate breast feeding to assist in natural placenta expulsion.

☐   If my doctor believes I am at risk of haemorrhaging, please allow the cord to stop pulsating before cutting. Then, please administer the pitocin/syntocinon for placenta delivery.

☐   Avoid pitocin/syntocinon unless there are any signs of hemorrhaging.

FOR BABY

We request:

- ☐ To have remove bright lights until baby is moved to mother's chest.
- ☐ Allow vernix to be absorbed into baby's skin; delay "cleaning or rubbing"; use soft cloth when rubbing is appropriate.
- ☐ Immediate skin to skin contact and delay procedures on baby
- ☐ Allow baby to remain with mother and/or birth companion for bonding
- ☐ Oral Vitamin K to be used if it is available (or)
- ☐ Delay Vitamin K injection until after baby is acclimatised
- ☐ Delay Hepatitis B injection until we see our GP (or)
- ☐ Delay Hepatitis B until later in our stay
- ☐ Father will stay with mother and baby throughout the hospital stay.
- ☐ Breast feeding several times during the first few hours after birth.
- ☐ Breast feeding only. No bottles, formula, dummies, artificial nipples.

We are planning a natural birth through hypnobirthing, yet we understand that birth can take a different direction for us. If this should happen; these are our requests:

IF A CAESAREAN BECOMES NECESSARY

We request:

- ☐ To be placed on a slightly raised angle to see more of the birth. *(45 degree angle to view and assist)*
- ☐ To have my birth music playing in the room.
- ☐ Please have quiet in the room and allow the baby to hear our voices first.
- ☐ To shield our baby from direct bright light (where possible)
- ☐ To assist in the delivery of our baby *(Once the baby's head/shoulders are visible and out I would like to be guided in placing my hands under the arms of my baby and assist in lifting the baby out of my stomach onto my chest)*
- ☐ To have sterile hands/gloves to assist in delivery *(to help prevent infection in case of contact with wound)*
- ☐ If unable to assist in the delivery, please place the baby on my chest immediately
- ☐ If my baby requires procedures (where possible), please perform these while by baby is at my chest.
- ☐ The baby to remain on my chest whist being stitched up.
- ☐ If the baby requires separation from mother, please allow father/birth partner to be with the baby at all times.
- ☐ Not to have a date set for a caesarean, but to allow our baby to come into the world on a date chosen by him/her. I will attend the hospital once my waters break or I start contractions whichever one comes first.

IF AN EPIDURAL BECOMES NECESSARY

We request:

☐   Please follow as much as the original birth plan as possible and advise me on changes.

☐   I would prefer a 'narcotic' or 'walking' epidural, so I can be more active in my birth and require less monitoring.

☐   I would like to be helped into a birthing position that uses gravity to aid the birth of my baby. If this is not possible, please allow me birth in the side lying position and support my top leg.

☐   Please turn down the epidural prior to the birthing stage, so I can gain feedback from my body in effective pushing.

☐   I have learnt the Hypnobirthing 'Perfect Pushing' for Interventions and I will only need minimal assistance with pushing.

Thank you for your support in advance to help us have a wonderful and fulfilling birth experience.

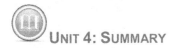

Unit 4: Summary

- Your body has the **imprinted knowledge** of how to give birth. Trust that innate ability and allow yourself to flow with each and every stage of your birthing time. Let go and allow your body to do its job.

- **Consider very carefully** if your body needs intervention in birthing, as each intervention can affect the course of your birth often in dramatic ways. Check to see if fear or real medical necessity is influencing your choice.

- **Being active in birth** and choosing the best birth positions will reduce your birthing time and bring additional comfort. Birth breathing will be easier, with less need for intervention.

- **Additional comfort measures** can be helpful in birthing, so add these to your tool kit, and on the birthing day you will have a wide range of effective natural comfort options.

- **Create your own Anesthesia for Birthing**, this is a very effective way of reducing or even eliminating strong sensations. Use the amazing power of your mind, and the 'Pain Gate Theory' to block sensations and birth in comfort.

- **Having a birth plan,** is a vital communication tool with your caregivers. Ensure everyone at your birth is familiar with your birth preferences.

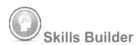

Skills Builder

- If you are listening the Hypnobirthing recording 'Creating Anesthesia for Birthing'. It is important to **stay awake** when listening to this recording to actively create the numbing feeling and then transfer it. (This is not one to listen to when you want to sleep).

- If you are practicing the anesthesia trigger, test to see how this works. Say 1,2,3,4 ....'numb' and feel your hand getting tingly and loosing sensations. Do this at a time when you don't have the benefit of the recording, as you will be able to create the 'numb' sensations on your own.

- Choose what birth positions you would like to be in at your birth. You may need to do more exercise and preparation (such as the squat) to accomplish them. Practice all your active birth exercises, so you are familiar with what to do for each stage on the day.

- Fill out your birth plan with your partner and then take to your caregiver as early as you can. This will enable you to quickly clear up any issues with your career and work towards your clarifying your choices. When this is done...visualize your amazing birthing day.

Partners Can Help

- Know all the stages of birth and what to do for each stage can make the difference in providing the best support.

- Trust her body, the same body that has worked perfectly to carry the baby in pregnancy to birth the baby just as well.

- Be familiar with the additional comfort measures before the birth and be proactive on the birthing day to know what to provide and when.

- Her body needs to be active to birth effectively, quickly and easily. Encourage her to stay off the bed as much as possible and assist her with the positions.

- Creating Anesthesia tool is very powerful and effective; if you are using this, practice this with her until you both know how to use it. You will be surprised how it can help with your own ailments.

I have the Knowledge: Checklist

☐ I know about the stages of my birth and I will be prepared for the wonderful day

☐ My body and my baby will let me know when it is the right time to be born. If I need help, I choose natural methods of induction first.

☐ If a hospital induction becomes necessary; I am confident of my choices and options

☐ Hypnobirthing provides comfort for natural births; if my birth has a change of plans and I require pain relief; I am aware of my best options.

☐ I know how to be active in my birth and choose the best birthing positions

☐ I am familiar with the many natural and alternative comfort measuring in birthing

☐ My birth partner and I are confident with Light Touch Massage

☐ My birth partner and I are confident with Counter Pressure Massage

☐ The Anesthesia Trigger in my tool box to use on the day of my birth, if I need it.

☐ I am confident that my birth plan is a good representation of my birth choices

Unit 3: Hypnobirthing Home Study Course Recordings

 Anesthesia for Easy Birthing

☐ T3 Creating Anesthesia for Birthing
Listen until you can recreate the triggers without the recording

 Rainbow Relaxation for Birth

☐ T1 Introduction
☐ T2 Rainbow Relaxation
☐ T3 Birthing Relaxation
☐ T4 Birth Partner Relax and be Confident *(for birth partners only)*
Listen to at least one relaxation each week until the birth

 Audio Guide – Unit 4 (Track 4)

This guide comprises of additional material to support Unit 4 of Hypnobirthing Home Study Course. You can listen once, or as many times as you need. The audio guide is the only recording that you can listen to while you are driving in the car. ***Podcast:*** *For this free audio track on this unit, go to* *http://hypnobirthinghub.podbean.com/ (Episode 5).*

 Videos: Hypnobirthing Techniques

Step by step guide to easily master the Hypnobirthing Hub techniques.
These video techniques App can be downloaded for free on both iTunes and Android.
Alternatively, these are also freely available on our website.
  • Counter Pressure Massage
  • Light Touch Massage

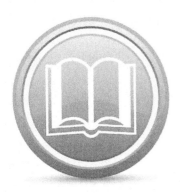

UNIT 5: REVIEW AND PRACTICE

Well done for completing the information units of the course. This unit is a summary and review, so it's time to see what you know and what you need to work on. With continued focus and practice of the Hypnobirthing Hub Home Study Course program, you will find that on the day of your birth, the tools and techniques will flow effortlessly and you begin to relax even more, with a confidence that this will indeed by an easy comfortable birth.

Hypnobirthing Home Study Course Foundations

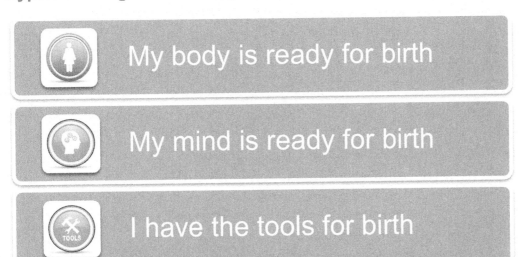

My body is ready for birth

My mind is ready for birth

I have the tools for birth

I have the knowledge for birth

MY BODY IS READY FOR BIRTH: WEEKLY EXERCISE EXAMPLE

	Monday	Tuesday	Wednesday	Thursday	Friday	Saturday	Sunday
		Pregnancy Relaxation and Health Mp3					
AM & PM - Teeth	Super Pelvic Floor 10 x 2	Super Pelvic Floor 10 x2	Super Pelvic Floor 10 x 2	Super Pelvic Floor 10 x 2	Super Pelvic Floor 10 x2	Super Pelvic Floor 10 x2	Super Pelvic Floor 10 x 2
Exercise: Yoga/ Pilates Swimming Walking							
Ball sitting Side to Side Hula Hoop Legs Wide							
Wall Squat							
Pelvic Rock							
Leg Press							
Leg Stretch							
Perineal Massage (35 weeks+)							

✔ I have seen a chiropractor/physiotherapist (pregnancy specialist); my pelvis and ligaments are ready for birth

✔ I am sitting correctly with supported chair or cross legged whenever I can

✔ I am consciously correcting my posture when standing and walking

This is just an example of a timetable to prepare your body for birth, please tailor your own schedule to your own preferences. Please continue with the exercises and preparation until your birthing day. In addition, many of these exercises will be part of your 'Active Birth' to help facilitate a shorter and easier birth for you and your baby.

My mind's ready for birth: checklist

- ☐ I am more aware of negative birth thoughts and how this affects my birth outlook.
- ☐ I understand how fear at birth causes Fear – Tension – Pain; I have done all I can to remove fear from my birthing day. I am looking forward to my birth.
- ☐ If I have a fear or unhelpful birth thought, I easily find the right emotional release tool
- ☐ I have protected my mind by only hearing positive birth stories, videos, TV where possible. I know my birth will be my own.
- ☐ Over time I am finding I have less need to monitor my negative thoughts, they are becoming more positive.
- ☐ I know the laws of the mind and I am choosing to use these to my advantage by preparing my mind for the best possible birth.
- ☐ I am confident in my birth can be one filled with positivity, joy and peace

EMOTIONAL RELEASE TOOLS

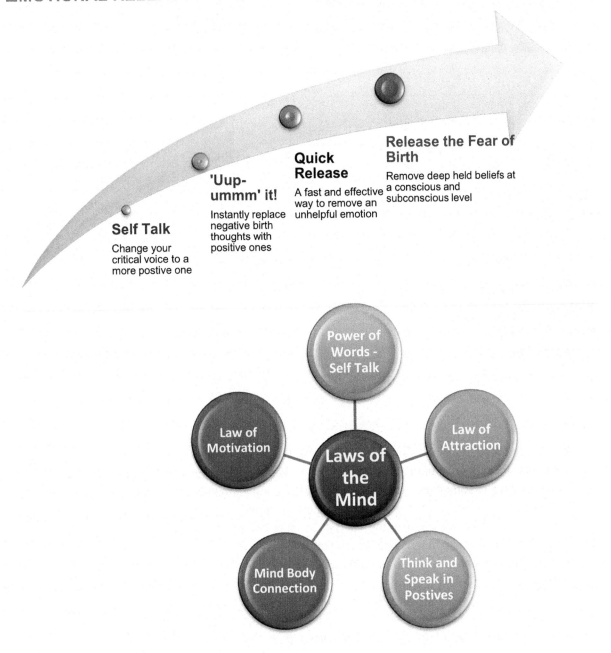

Release the Fear of Birth
Remove deep held beliefs at a conscious and subconscious level

Quick Release
A fast and effective way to remove an unhelpful emotion

'Uup-ummm' it!
Instantly replace negative birth thoughts with positive ones

Self Talk
Change your critical voice to a more postive one

Power of Words - Self Talk

Law of Motivation

Laws of the Mind

Law of Attraction

Mind Body Connection

Think and Speak in Postives

I HAVE THE TOOLS FOR BIRTH

The Hypnobirthing Breathing

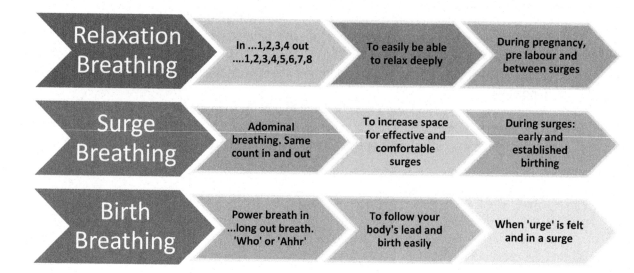

The Hypnobirthing Triggers

Relaxation Trigger	1,2,3,4....relax	Hand on shoulder (upon 'relax')	Deepens your relaxation
Relaxation Trigger (Special Place)	1,2,3,4....relax	Transports you to your special place	Connected to your baby during surges
Quick Release Trigger	1,2,3,4 ...release	Long out breath on 'release'	Feel the emotion releasing
Anesthesia Trigger (Hand Numb)	(1,2,3,4 ...numb)	Hand becoming numb	Hand removed of sensations
Anesthesia Trigger (Transferring)	1,2,3,4 ...release	Place numb hand on body. Long out breath on 'release'	Feel the numbness releasing to the body; for comfortable birthing

I have the tools for birth: checklist

- ☐ Relaxation breathing is easy and I use it anytime I need to find peace and calm
- ☐ Surge breathing is becoming automatic and 'my balloon' is continually rising up higher
- ☐ Birth breathing is something I am comfortable with practice daily from 35 weeks
- ☐ Perfect pushing (intervention) is practiced in case a 'change of plans' is needed
- ☐ My partner and I are confident in the 1,2,3,4,....Relax Trigger
- ☐ My partner and I are confident with Touch Relaxation
- ☐ I have a special place to use when I am in a surge
- ☐ I visualize my perfect birth often
- ☐ I see the 'Baby Head Down' and 'Butterfly from Cocoon' pictures daily
- ☐ I use the Quick Release Trigger: 1,2,3,4 ....release, to gain emotional freedom
- ☐ The Anesthesia Triggers are working and I will birth in comfort

I HAVE THE KNOWLEDGE FOR BIRTH

Use your BRAIN for a change of plans

BRAIN

B Benefits

R Risks

A Alternative

I Intuition

N Nothing (at least for a while)

I have the knowledge for birth: checklist

- ☐ I know about the stages of my birth and I will be prepared for the wonderful day.
- ☐ My birth plan reflects my choices and my caregiver is supportive of my plan.
- ☐ My body and my baby will let me know when it is the right time to be born. If I need help, I choose natural methods of induction first.
- ☐ If a hospital induction becomes necessary; I am confident of my choices.
- ☐ Hypnobirthing provides comfort for natural births; if my birth has a change of plans and I require pain relief; I am aware of my best options.
- ☐ I know how to be active in my birth and choose the best birthing positions.
- ☐ I am familiar with the array of natural and alternative comfort measuring in birthing.
- ☐ My birth partner and I are confident with light touch massage.
- ☐ My birth partner and I are confident with counter pressure massage.
- ☐ The Anesthesia Triggers are in my tool box to use on the day of my birth.

Hypnobirthing Home Study Course Recordings

For some mothers reading this section, may have many months before the wonderful birthing day arrives and for some others it could be a precious few weeks away. Therefore, wherever relevant I have indicated what to focus on before and after thirty-five weeks. Your Hypnobirthing success is not an equation based on the amount of recordings you listen nor the amount of practice you do. And so this section below is just a guide for you. Some mothers will do more, particularly just prior to birth and some mothers will birth beautifully with much less effort. You will know what the right amount of listening and Hypnobirthing practice is for you. The checklists are a more accurate gauge of your Hypnobirthing skills and confidence. If there is anything that you are unsure of, take the time to go over the relevant section once more. Your mind/body and your baby are counting on you!

 Part 1 - Pregnancy Relaxation and Health

    T1 Introduction
    T2 Pregnancy Relaxation and Health
    T3 Quick Relaxation and Baby Bonding
    T4 Pregnancy Affirmations

Listen to the tracks **regularly** from now until the birth of your baby. By listening to these recordings consistently, it will provide the best possible pregnancy experience for you and be a simple reminder for continued health and relaxation during your pregnancy.

***Before* 35 weeks:** *Listen to at least two tracks once per week. You may like to focus more on this recording and less on the other Hypnobirthing Hub recordings.*

__After__ 35 weeks: Listen to at least one track each week and then focus your attention on the other Hypnobirthing Hub recordings.

Part 2 - Release all Fear of Birth
T1 Introduction
T2 Release the Fear of Birth
T3 Quick Release – Fear
T4 Quick Release – Problems
T5 Quick Release – Relationship

Listen **once** to T2 Release the Fear of Birth. This is a long therapy session to remove deep fears or unhelpful beliefs about birth. Listen again if needed. The Quick Release tracks are an aid in finding emotional freedom when issues arise.

Part 3 - Rainbow Relaxation for Birth
T1 Introduction
T2 Rainbow Relaxation
T3 Birthing Relaxation
T4 Birth Partner Relax and be Confident (birth partners only)

These tracks are perfect to listen to as you go off to sleep, just pick one to listen to as you drift off. The Rainbow Relaxation is designed for both partners as it is a general relaxation with minimal birth content in it. The Birth Partner Relaxation is only for birth partners and is an excellent summary of what to do on the birthing day.

Mothers: Listen to T2 Rainbow Relaxation and T3 Birthing Relaxation once per week.
Partners: Listen to T4 Birth Partner Relax and T2 Rainbow Relaxation once per week.

Part 4 - Breathing and Birth Visualisation
T1 Introduction
T2 Visualise your Amazing Birth
T3 Birth Affirmations
T4 Relaxation Breathing
T5 Surge Breathing (Contractions)
T6 Birth Breathing

Listen to these tracks once a week until the birth. T2 Visualise and T3 Birthing Affirmations can be listened to as you fall asleep or Listen to Birthing Affirmations while getting ready in the morning.

__Before__ 35 weeks: Focus on learning the breathing techniques.
__After__ 35 weeks: Increase your breathing practice until it is automatic. Practice relaxation and Surge Breathing (with or without the recording) every day for five minutes each. Practice your Birth Breathing each time you do a bowel movement.

Part 5 - Anesthesia for Easy Birthing
T1 Introduction
T2 Relaxation Triggers and Special Place
T3 Creating Anesthesia for Birthing

These are the more advanced Hypnobirthing techniques and are very helpful to create deep relaxation and comfortable birthing. Make sure you are **sitting upright and awake** to get the best use out of these tracks.

Mothers: Listen to T2 Relaxation Triggers **once** to create the trigger. Practice the Relaxation Triggers once a week and throughout the day whenever you need it. Listen again as needed to deepen the trigger. Listen to T3 Creating Anesthesia **once per week** and practice the Anesthesia Triggers **once per week**.

Birth Partners: Listen to T2 Relaxation Triggers **once** to create the trigger. Practice the Relaxation Triggers with your partner (your hand on her shoulder) **once per week**. Listen again to T2 to deepen the trigger.

 Part 6 - Your Birthing Day Guide
T1 Introduction
T2 Early Comfortable Birthing
T3 Moving to your Birthing Place
T4 Established Comfortable Birthing
T5 Birthing – Breathe your Baby out
T6 Quick Release – Change of Plans

These recording are a helpful summary of Hypnobirthing Home Study Course and are designed to be listened for each stage of your birthing day. It will calm and remind you of the tools, techniques and stages of birth. This is a must to bring at the birth!

Before 35 weeks: Some women have found it helpful to listen once before 35 weeks.
After 35 weeks: Listen **once per week** and take these recordings with you to your birth.

 Part 7 – Audio Guide
T1 Introduction
T2 Unit 1
T3 Unit 2
T4 Unit 3
T5 Unit 4

These instructional recordings are designed to accompany Hypnobirthing Home Study Course material. Listen to the audio guide at least once or as many times as you like. These are the only Hypnobirthing recordings that can be listened to while driving or operating machinery.
Tip: If you are finding it difficult to persuade your birth partner to read the manual, these recordings are an easy way to introduce Hypnobirthing.

Part 8 - Birth Music

T1 Introduction
T2 Pure Embrace
T3 Adrift
T4 Sea waves

These T2 and T3 are the background music in all Hypnobirthing Home Study Course recordings. By listening to these tracks regularly provides an audio relaxation trigger. It will also subconsciously remind you of Hypnobirthing Home Study Course material on the day of your birth. This recording is a must to take to your birthing place. Many women find T4 Sea waves, helpful in creating a gentle rhythm in their Surge Breathing.

Hypnobirthing Home Study Course: Review Guide

Key Points

- **This is a weekly** practice and review guide. Continue with the suggested guide until thirty-five weeks. After this time, swap to *'Review After 35 Weeks'*
- **This is just a guide**; you will know what is right for you.
  - If you started your Hypnobirthing practice early in your pregnancy you may choose to do less after thirty-five weeks
  - If you started your Hypnobirthing practice later in your pregnancy you may choose to do more after thirty-five weeks
- **Relaxation is the key** to your Hypnobirthing success. Create the habit of relaxing every day.
- Many of the tracks can be listened to **while going to sleep**; and so create an effective use of time.
- **Visualization is important** as is prepares your mind for a good birth outcome and 'cements' the new more positive beliefs about birth.
- **Hypnobirthing breathing is a vital part** of creating relaxation and comfort in the birth stages. Practice these until you are confident in your ability to automatically recall them at birth.
- **The hypnobirthing Tools** are a quick and easy way of gaining relaxation, emotional release and comfort. Practice until you are confident in their use.
- **Partner Practice regularly** will strengthen the tools and techniques learnt. It will also give you both confidence in your new Hypnobirthing abilities, so on the day of birth you will feel supported, have greater trust, connection to each other and your birthing goals.
- **Exercise is important:** remember to continue to follow 'My Body is Ready for Birth' examples
- Have you finished the **Skills Builder Exercises** for Units 1 -4?
- Have you finished the **Unit 1 to 4 listening** of the following?
  - Release all Fear of Birth
  - Audio Guide (Units 1-4)
  - Relaxation Triggers and Special Place

Hypnobirthing Hub Home Study Course

Review Weekly Example (Before 35 weeks)

	Monday	Tuesday	Wednesday	Thursday	Friday	Saturday	Sunday
Relaxation	T2 Pregnancy Relaxation and Health	T2 Rainbow Relaxation	T3 Quick Relaxation and Baby Bonding		T3 Birth Relaxation		
Visualisation	T4 Pregnancy Affirmations (Visualise)		Go to 'Special Place' and visualise your birth			T2. Visualise your Amazing Birth	T3 Birth Affirmations (Visualise)
Breathing		Practice Surge and Relaxation Breathing		Breathing Tracks			
Other Hypnobirthing				Birth Music with own relaxation			T3 Creating Anesthesia
Tools	Practice Relaxation Triggers		Practice Quick Release Triggers		Practice Anesthesia Triggers		
Partner Practice		Relaxation Trigger (partner hand on her shoulder)		Light touch and counter pressure massages			Partner Directed Touch Relaxation
Birth Partner		T2 Rainbow Relaxation				T4 Birth Partner Relaxation	

☐   I am continuing with the 'Prepare my Body for Birth' exercises.

Hypnobirthing Hub Home Study Course
Review Weekly Example (After 35 weeks)

	Monday	Tuesday	Wednesday	Thursday	Friday	Saturday	Sunday
Relaxation	T2 Pregnancy Relaxation and Health or T3 Quick Relaxation	T2 Rainbow Relaxation			T3 Birth Relaxation		
Visualisation	T3 Birth Affirmations (Visualise)		Go to 'Special Place' and visualise your birth			T2. Visualise your Amazing Birth	T3 Birth Affirmation (Visualise)
Breathing	Practice Relaxation and Surge Breathing every day. Practice Birth Breathing with each bowel movement.						
Other Hypnobirthing			Your Birthing Day Guide Recording	Birth Music with own relaxation			T3 Creating Anesthesia
Tools	Practice Relaxation Triggers		Practice Quick Release Triggers		Practice Anesthesia Triggers		
Partner Practice		Relaxation Trigger (partner hand on her shoulder)		Light touch and counter pressure massages			Partner Directed Touch Relaxation
Birth Partner		T2 Rainbow Relaxation				T4 Birth Partner Relaxation	

- ☐ I see the 'Baby Head Down' and 'Butterfly from Cocoon' pictures daily.
- ☐ I am continuing with the 'Prepare my Body for Birth' exercises.

Note: If you are completing Hypnobirthing Home Study Course later in your pregnancy, you may wish to increase your weekly listening and practice.

THE DAY OF YOUR BIRTH – SUMMARY AND GUIDE

PRE LABOR WARM UPS

Listen to your choice of Hypnobirthing Hub Home Study Course Recordings.

Body

- Cervix softens and ripens, thins out, and starts to open slightly (or dilate) up to about one to three centimetres.
- Some physical signs the birthing time could be starting.
- Practice surges can occur from a few week or days prior to the birth, or on the actual birthing day.

Active- pre labor

- As much rest as possible. The more you sleep and allow your body to do the work for you, the faster this time will pass.
- Do not get into your birthing mode. Your body is working behind the scenes. Rest where you can or keep busy by going for a walk or some easy exercises.
- Keep well-nourished and hydrated to maintain good energy levels to help you birth your baby.

Mind

- Birth takes as long as it takes. Your body knows what to do; let go and trust it to get on with the job.
- Focus on the positive; you've waited nine months, and only a little longer.
- Monitor your birth self-talk, it is important to be confident in this stage.
- Need to do a Quick Release of any issues that arise?

Tools

- Relaxation breathing when you need it to provide a sense of calm and comfort.
- Only a few minutes of Surge Breathing when you feel pre labor warm up surges, to gain some practice for your birthing time.

Knowledge

- If you are unsure if this is the 'real deal', there is no harm in visiting place of birth or calling your caregiver for peace of mind.
- For strong and lengthy pre labor warm ups, check for unusual positions. It's the body's way of preparing muscles and pelvis for a more challenging birth.

Birth Partners

- Provide all the comfort, attention and understanding in this delicate 'waiting game'.
- Keep yourself busy at this time and go about your normal routine, while being easily contactable if things progress.
- It is also a great time to practice comfort measure techniques.
- Provide to her the encouragement that you know the Hypnobirthing Tools and Techniques.

EARLY BIRTHING TIME

Listen to 'Your Birthing Day Guide' Track 2 'Early Confident Birthing'.

Body

Early birthing surges often start, build up to a peak, and then fade away. Surges become more regular about five minutes apart, lasting for approximately 40-45 seconds.

- This change can be obvious; with surges stronger, longer and frequent. For others, the change is less noticeable.
- The cervix is very thin and opens (or dilates) to four centimetres.

Active early birthing

- Be active only some of the time, you need rest.
- If surges at night, sleep or rest between surges with side lying or sitting upright.
- Sitting upright, standing and walking positions are best options for early birthing helping surges become regular and rhythmic.
- Sitting and movement on the exercise ball encourages rhythmic movement and pelvic mobility.

Mind

- Protect yourself from becoming overwhelmed by the sights, sounds and seriousness of birth. Remember your emotional release tools.
- We know of the delicate hormonal balance and the effect of adrenaline can have on birthing.
- Remember to stay at home as long as you feel comfortable doing so.
- Start out how you wish to go on. The more relaxed, comfortable, and at ease with your surges at this stage, will lay the foundation for an easy established birthing.

Tools

- Effective surge breathing will provide the best source of relaxation at this stage and will make the surges more effective and less intense.
- During surges: go to your special place, relax fully and focus on your surge breathing. You may like to;
    - Sit on a chair with your head against a pillow
    - On all fours with your head resting against an exercise ball
    - Relax in a bath or shower (sitting down)
    - Sit on a recliner with a pillow for your head
- Most Hypnobirthing mothers find this stage very manageable and even easy.

Knowledge

- First baby: the early birthing time can take some time; so spend this time at home. Contact your birth partner to be to support you.
- Second and subsequent baby: often significantly reducing this phase and more quickly. Calmly move to your birthing place when you feel ready to go.

Birth Partners

- In a surge there is a 'no talk' rule for you and the caregivers
- Between surges she is mostly her usual self and will rely on you to provide conversation and interaction.
- It is your calm and confident manner that will have the most impact upon your partner's relaxation and state of mind. Treasure this role.
- Clearly demonstrate to her, your solid belief in her ability to birth calmly, safely and easily. Your encouragement will make all the difference.

ESTABLISHED BIRTHING TIME

Listen to 'Your Birthing Day Guide' Track 3 'Moving to your Birth Place' and Track 4 'Established Comfortable Birthing'.

Body

- Past the four centimetres hurdle as your cervix will now be quickly opening, as the softening and thinning is usually completed.

- Your cervix is opening from four to eight centimetres.
- Your body is working very hard now to open up your cervix. The surges are strong to achieve this.
- Surges are often 45-60 seconds long and 3-5 minutes apart.

Active - established birthing

- This is the most important stage to be active; to aid pelvic mobility and baby's assent into the pelvis.
- Use your choice of active birth positions and exercises. Importantly stay off the bed and when sitting keep your feet on the floor.
- Choose some active positions that expose your back for your partner to provide massage or relaxation techniques
- If tired and bed seems like the best place to be, use pillows or wedges to lie down on your side. Remember that surges are more intense in laying down positions.

Mind

- Your awareness naturally goes inward and becomes more primal at this time.
- Between surges; a dreaminess and time warping appears.
- You become totally absorbed and not want to be disturbed. Let go and allow your body to do its job.
- Think 'primal'; create a quiet, dark, warm, and safe environment.
- Deep relaxation is the key to your comfortable surges. The more relaxed you are the easier they will be.
- Your needs change rapidly; your birth partner will adjust accordingly.

Tools

- Surges are getting more powerful and you may need some extra comfort measures.
- Concentrate deeply on your surge breathing. Use your relaxation trigger to go to your special place with each surge.
- Use different hypnobirthing tools, triggers, massages, and additional comfort measures.
- Counter pressure massage can make a big difference during a surge.

Knowledge

- Move to the place of your birth when you feel ready. This stage can last for many hours, particularly for first time mothers.
- To bring additional comfort to a surge – lift your bottom and leaning forward with the surge.
- Some find it helpful to rock with each surge while leaning forwards and straightening up in between surges.

Birth Partner

- You are the keeper and enforcer of the birth plan. Ensure all caregivers understand your birth choices.
- If changes arise, ask caregivers to speak with you first. Then think B.R.A.I.N
- Deep relaxation is the key to comfortable surges. It is important that you do all you can to encourage the deepest level of relaxation.
- Create a 'primal' environment; a quiet, dark, warm, and safe environment, the more she can birth like a mammal, the better.
- She usually has an accurate sense of 'when it is time' to leave for the hospital or birth centre. Have trust in her instincts. She will only labor well if she is feeling at ease, and in control of the decisions.
- Her needs change rapidly; be prepared for this, and adjust the comfort measure or approach accordingly.

- Her awareness naturally goes inward and becomes more primal at this time and is totally absorbed and may not want any interaction with you for the moment.
- Between surges; a dreaminess and time warping appears. She is less likely to want general conversation.

TRANSITION STAGE

Listen to your Birth Music at this stage to provide comfort and relaxation.

Body

- Around eight to ten centimetres dilation, the uterus has a burst of energy to quickly get ready for birthing.
- Stage is very short; five to thirty minutes, before surges rest and the body prepares for birthing.
- Surges become more intense and sometimes extremely powerful.
- Surges are sixty to ninety seconds long with two minutes apart.
- Physical signs your body is working really hard – hot and cold flushes, shaking, nausea, and vomiting. These are normal physical responses to hard work.

Active - transition

- Being upright at this stage is vital to allow the bones and ligaments of the pelvis to move and adjust to ease the passage for the baby.
- If sitting, feet must be on the floor for best pelvic mobility.
- No active exercises needed at this time; get into the most comfortable position for surges.
- After transition, there is break from surges. It's important to stay in the upright position to facilitate an easy decent for the baby.

Mind

- It can be a time when you suddenly feel that you are unsure that you will be able to carry on and begin to doubt yourself.
- This stage is so short; it could be over in five minutes.
- Some mothers start to think a little irrationally and believe they can leave their birthing.
- Some mothers don't actually experience an increase in discomfort during this stage, but they do feel their emotions have changed.
- This phase is normal and is an indication of your good progression and close to having your baby. This can be very reassuring.
- Once 'the urge' appears; self-doubt goes. You become energised, determined and focused in birthing your baby.

Tools

- Surges are getting more powerful and you may need some extra comfort measures.
- Counter pressure massage works well at this stage.
- Relaxation Trigger and Touch Relaxation is beneficial to increase relaxation.
- The best 'tool' is the reassurance from your birth partner.

Knowledge

- This is the time to really relax and just ride with it. Take each surge for what it is, and focus only on the present moment.
- Remember, at all times, that you are simply experiencing a feeling, a sensation within your body that you can work with. It can be intense, hard and challenging, but can also be incredible and truly empowering.
- Some mothers don't have any noticeable transitional period.
- This phase is only short and leads to a resting phase. You could be holding your baby in your arms in fifteen minutes to two hours.

Birth Partner

- Transition phase is normal and to be expected, both she and the baby are OK and doing what nature intended.
- It will be easier from here, not harder. If she been free from medical pain relief up until this point, then she will not need it now.
- Encourage her into an upright position.
- Listen attentively to her breathing. You may now have to control the speed of breathing, slow it down, and really concentrate on ensuring her body is really relaxed and limp.
- She may not want too much attention or comfort measures at this time, or she will be very specific about what she does want! Support her with your patience and understanding.
- This is the time to really encourage and praise her. Let her know that she is soon going to give birth to a wonderful baby and coming close to the end.
- After transition, there is break between the surges, encourage her to stay in the upright position to facilitate an easy decent for the baby.

BIRTHING STAGE

Listen to 'Your Birthing Day Guide' Track 5 Birthing your Baby or Birth Music playing on loud speaker.

Body

- The cervix is fully open; the **hormone relaxin** helps the muscles in the birth canal to open. These muscles can spread out and expand to be large enough for a baby to pass through.
- The body steps up a gear and the longitudinal muscles begin to push the baby down into the birth canal.
- Once the baby is around two centimetres into the birth canal, this urge to bear down, or "foetal ejection reflex" occurs.
- By trusting your body and allowing the urge to bear down to come naturally, your body will do the rest.

Active - Birthing

- Squatting is the **most beneficial birth position** in that it opens the pelvis wide, shortens the birth canal and uses gravity to encourage the baby to descend. This position is known to shorten the birthing phase of labor.
- Choose positions that make use of gravity, for an easier decent.
- If your baby is very big or in a posterior position, you may like to birth on your hand and knees.

Mind

- All self-doubt is removed and is replaced with determination and focus. You now are energised and ready to birth, as your body receives a much needed energy boost at this time.
- This stage can be over in five to thirty minutes, it won't be long now.
- If you have birthed well up until this point, then it is smooth sailing from here on end. It is unlikely there will be the need for intervention.

Tools

- Once the urge is there; your focus should be on listening to your body, following your 'Birth Breathing' and going with the sensations - your body will do the rest. Now is the time to trust your body.
- It is important not to be hurried into pushing, as research has shown that forced pushing brings many negatives to mother and baby.

- Remember the butterfly and cocoon visualization picture, slow down your decent of birthing your baby. It will happen naturally as you allow your baby to rest on your perineum until it is stretched enough for your baby's head to pass through.

Knowledge

- Once the baby has moved down through the birth canal, the muscles of the perineum gradually flatten out and cover a much wider area just as the baby is coming out.
- The pressure of the baby's head on the perineum reduces circulation, which helps to numb the area.
- The cells of the perineum have more elasticity than any other part of the body and are flooded with the hormone relaxin to enable them to fan open in order to allow the baby to pass through.

Birth Partner

- Your job is almost over, and there is not much to do here except provide all the encouragement she will need to birth her baby.
- Many women will want their hands held as they birth the baby; it is a way of gaining support and also greeting the new baby together into the world.
- Have your T-shirt ready for some skin to skin time with the new baby.
- Remember to monitor the birth choices in cutting the cord and delivering the placenta.

Take pride in knowing you chose to give you and your baby the best possible birth experience. We wish you happiness, joy, love and laughter as you welcome your ray of sunshine into the world.

Resources and Free Hypnobirthing

Join the thousands of women around the world, who had the most amazing birth experiences. These women were comfortable, empowered and proud to birth naturally like so many before them. There is every reason that you can also birth with the power and wisdom of Hypnobirthing.

Mp3/Album Pack - Hypnobirthing Home Study Course

This series of eight albums/Mp3 will complement the knowledge you gained through the Hypnobirthing Home Study Course Manual. These albums are focused on creating a deeper experience of Hypnosis and relaxation to support you throughout your pregnancy and birth. You can download these individually or as a pack through our website **www.hypnobirthinghub.com/shop** alternatively they can be purchased through Amazon or ITunes.

Website: www.hypnobirthinghub.com

Blog Page: Regular blog posts of birth stories, videos, new findings and key information.

Resourses Page: Download birth plans and other important information.

Video Techniques: Step by step free videos demonstrating:

- Relaxation Breathing
- Surge Breathing
- Birth Breathing
- Perfect Pushing (for intervention)
- Light Touch Massage
- Comfort Pressure Massage

Also download these Hypnobirthing Video Techniques on a <u>free App</u> on iTunes or Android.

 Free Mp3: Pregnancy Health and Relaxation

Podcast

Discover a series of six free podcasts; giving more insight and depth to the Hypnobirthing Hub Home Study Course material. **http://hypnobirthinghub.podbean.com/**

Social Hypnobirthing

 https://www.facebook.com/hypnobirthinghub/

 Hypnobirthing Hub

 YouTube Channel: Hypnobirthing Hub

 https://twitter.com/HypnoBirthHub

 https://au.pinterest.com/hypnobirthinghub/

CPSIA information can be obtained
at www.ICGtesting.com
Printed in the USA
LVOW02s0549271016

510469LV00023B/454/P